Cancer, then no cancer

CANCER,
then
no cancer

A Handbook for Health and Healing

Liz Gamble AA, MA, NHC, Min.

Xulon Press

CancerThenNoCancer.com

Xulon Press
2301 Lucien Way #415
Maitland, FL 32751
407.339.4217
www.xulonpress.com

Printed in the United States of America.

ISBN-13: 9781545619650

Table of Contents

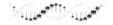

Cancer . . . then no cancer

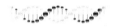

T his book is the story of how I changed my life and overcame breast cancer using natural alternative methods. It is a manual for good health and prevention of disease.

Preface

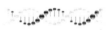

I would like to introduce myself and let you know the purpose of this book. In December of 2007, I was diagnosed with multi-foci breast cancer, but after the medical community gave me such frightening options, I chose not to accept their medical solution. I chose to listen to a Higher Power—Father God.

Up to this point, I had somewhat of an uneventful life, growing up in a middle-class family, probably a lot like yours. Throughout my career as an adult, my jobs had never been considered dangerous or environmentally hazardous. In fact, I was quite healthy my entire life, except for the common cold. I've never even suffered from a broken bone!

That was, until December 27, 2007, when I knew I was faced with the fight of my life. Sitting in the surgeon's office, I heard his words ringing through the cold, sterile office: It doesn't look good, Ms. Gamble. When

I looked at your biopsy, I found a substantial amount of cancer in the right breast. It isn't a lump or a tumor, but it looks like a string of pearls, which makes it impossible to operate to remove it. My only suggestion is a double mastectomy—nothing else will work—not even chemo or radiation. We won't know if the lymph nodes were affected until you have the surgery, but they may have to be removed too."

There was a long pause, but I finally mustered the courage to reply, "I am not scared to die; I am a Christian and My Creator must have a better report than what you just gave me. He knows me better than I know myself, so, I'm going to get a second opinion." I left his office, stating emphatically that I was not going to schedule the surgery. Who said there were no other options? The nurse offered me a few obligatory pamphlets on breast cancer and the phone numbers of some local support groups sponsored by the National Cancer Society.

Since that day, nothing in my life has been the same. My thoughts and feelings about what I thought was important, my lifestyle, everything was turned upside down, but the truth of the matter is it probably was right-side-up for the first time ever.

I'd like to tell you about this frightening, yet amazing year that followed this diagnosis because I believe, if it was possible for me to be healed, it's possible for you to discover that there are other healing options apart from your doctor's report. My journey began with the surgeon's report, but one year later, God turned what was meant for death into life. I feel the best — mentally, physically, and spiritually than I have ever imagined, and I believe there is hope and life for anyone who reads this book. As your health improves, I encourage you to share your success in this fight against cancer with others who are also in the battle, so you will begin to be a network of support.

"Man will realize that sickness of the soul is just as significant as the sickness of the body."

Louis Pasteur

Foreword

"I am persuaded, beyond all doubt, that neither death
nor life, nor angels nor principalities,
nor things present or impending and threatening,
nor things to come,
nor powers, nor height nor depth,
nor anything else in all creation
that will be able to separate me from the Love of God,
which is in Christ Jesus our Lord." Romans 8:38

"All things work together for the good,
to those who love God and are called
according to His design and purpose."
Romans 8:28

"And the fact that I am called to go through something that I don't like, and never planned on,
only allows tso perform on the center stage of my life
and to show off His Love and Glory. As I overcome, I
get stronger and I am set free. Now, I can share the road
for others to follow."

The Author

Introduction

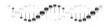

It's funny how life can throw you a curve when you least suspect it. Seems like everything is going along just the way you think it's supposed to, and WHAM! Here comes a bad report from the doctor! You look back through your personal files for "How do I get through this one?" and you can't seem to find your "Instructions to Life Book" . . . isn't everyone supposed to have one? But, at this point, you can't find the answers anywhere. These were my thoughts as I looked frantically for some way to get out of this. I was devastated; this was the most extreme report I had ever received.

However, from somewhere down in the innermost depths of my being came a cry. It was a loud cry, but a simple cry, "Help me, God! What is happening here? How in the world did this catastrophe sneak into my life?" Then, from an even deeper place, a stronger voice replied, "I've been waiting for you to ask Me." I knew the familiar sound of that voice that I was not alone. Peace swept over my spirit, and I knew everything would be all right. I didn't know exactly how it was going to happen, but I knew I wasn't in this by myself. And you aren't either.

Later that same voice told me that if I would devote one year, He would totally and completely heal me of this disease called breast cancer. I would come out with much, much more than I could have ever imagined. I have come to trust in that Love that was so freely given to me, and my whole life has forever changed.

I am healed and at peace with the world around me. There is a purpose for me to be on this planet, and I found mine through this pathway that the Father laid out for me.

I held onto His promise for the entire year, and now I can see everything better. In this hands-on manual, I want to share the process, the victory over cancer and how so much good can come from so much agony and fear. I want you to find the direction for your healing and recovery, and find a happy, healthy way to live life. Fasten your seatbelts because there is never a dull moment with God. All things are possible with Him.

For you, the reader, I pray complete healing and complete health over you and your family. I know you have probably already told your friends and family about your cancer diagnosis, but now you have a book to assist you in fighting the disease. Realize that victory won't come without sacrifice, and definitely not without some change, but we are building faith and trust in the Father with every step we take forward.

This is not a complicated walk; in fact, it's rather easy. I wrote this book to encourage you and to let you know that you will never be alone. If you've come to that place of despair, and you want some information that will be beneficial to you, this book will be your go-to manual. It will give you the information you need, so you can proudly walk through any indecision and confusion that is going on with you.

Maybe you are even in a depression and you've lost all hope because you think there is no place to turn. The doctors' reports are dismal, and the surgeons and the National Cancer Society keeps giving you the same worn-out news. Here, in this book, I have laid out a path of recovery that is more tangible and more positive than most of the 'surviving cancer' groups. I was told to write down the process exactly as I lived it, and there is hope for you. There is much that the doctors and the American Cancer Society haven't told you, but read on, and, hopefully, you'll see the Truth.

Another Option

I'd like to give you another option to the typical AMA prognosis, but it will involve answering some tough questions about yourself. I will ask you to examine the ways you have been eating that has caused you these problems; I will walk with you through whatever is required with peace instead of fear, and all I ask is that you keep an open mind. You have exceptional alternatives with this information, and it will flow like a river in the desert. While everyone around you is circulating clouds of death and negativity, this will be your life-line. I received complete healing without chemicals, radiation, or surgery because I took alternative information that I had researched and applied it to my circumstances. After I was declared cancer-free, I compiled everything into this one book. One resource for you to have.

This handbook will help you regain your sanity as well. It is my story, and I think you'll be able to relate to it easily, and, more importantly, it worked! I am one of many who have allowed the body to heal itself. Anyone who reads this book and applies the suggestions will be able to combat the disease of cancer plus other chronic diseases while also actively preventing disease. This book looks at the fact that all diseases have roots in the spiritual, mental, and physical parts of the person, and if one part is diseased, then all parts are affected. In order to recover completely, all three areas must be healed or the disease will continue to return.

For this reason, you could also use the components of the program to prevent oncoming diseases, strengthen your immune system, and improve your general health. Regardless of whether you've been diagnosed with cancer or you are using these methods for prevention, this book gives you ways to improve the quality of your life, while helping you build a healthy, nutritious new lifestyle of good health and energy. Really, becoming cancer-free is the bonus!

The bottom line is this: If we Americans would fight for our health like we fight for the remote, we would all be healthy and disease-free, but that's not the case. As you read the chapters and relate to the emotions and struggles I've gone through, you will slowly begin to unravel the knot that cancer has created in your soul. You'll find that this catastrophe will present a platform for you to reach higher than you ever thought possible, even though it looked like there was no hope.

Short story: Fear knocked at the door, and Faith answered. There was no one there. Faith wins!

There is no time in God, so put your watch and cal-endar away. When your report comes back clear, and you find yourself in the best health ever, like many have done, you will have learned an important lesson in life: always get the second opinion. You'll soon find that you're in the middle of a life so full of possibilities that you'll never look back to the lifestyle that got you in this position. You'll always be moving forward.

This is my story and I want to share it with you, so you too can find the road to recovery. May God Bless you and guide you as you read and get involved. The nutritional plan in chapter 5 -7 is the heart of the recovery, but the essence and actions of the other chapters are equally as important. Getting started right away is the best idea. Read, relate, and concede to your innermost being to what recovery really sounds like. It'll be music to your ears.

The Winning Results

```
Chk-in #   Order   Exam      Description
3584044    0001    16070     CW MM DIAG MAMMO DIGITAL BIL
                             Ord Diag: 793.80-AB MAMMOGRAM NOS
                             CPT/MOD: G0204

DOS: 07/22/08 1335                                    FINAL


   BILATERAL DIAGNOSTIC MAMMOGRAM

   Craniocaudal and mediolateral oblique views of both breasts are compared
   to a previous study of June 22, 2007 and May 8, 2006.

   Patient is status post two right breast biopsies, the most recent being
   in December 2007, at the more posterior side, which revealed invasive
   lobular carcinoma. This is a new postbiopsy baseline for the right
   breast which shows some minimal scarring near the area in question and
   no new focal suspicious mass or clustered microcalcification.

   IMPRESSION:

   Stable left breast. New baseline established for right breast, following
   new diagnosis in December 2007. Recommend six month followup of the
   right breast in the perioperative period.

   BI-RADS 3

   This examination was reviewed with the aid of CAD.

   PLEASE NOTE:  -----------------------------------------------------

   A.  A negative x-ray report should not delay biopsy if a dominant or
   clinically suspicious mass is present. Ten percent of cancers are not
   identified by x-ray.
   B.  A negative report may reinforce clinical impressions.
   C.  Adenosis and dense breasts may obscure an underlying neoplasm.
   D.  False positive reports average 6%-10%.
                   Thank you for your referral!
--------------------------------------------------------------------
C:;SHEPARD,DEBORAH K:SHEPARD,DEBORAH K:335 CLYDE MORRIS BLVD;SUITE 240;ORMOND BE
                              PT: GAMBLE,ELIZABETH K
                              BD: 10/15/57   Age: 50Y   Sex: F
          SHEPARD,DEBORAH K       DOS: 07/22/08 1335      MR #: C000175026
          335 CLYDE MORRIS BLVD   LOC: DIS - COP
          ORMOND BEACH, FL 32174  PCP DR:
                              ADM DR: SHEPARD,DEBORAH K
   Print Date/Time: 07/23/08 0817   UNK          Page  CONTINUED *
```

Chapter 1

The Enemy and the Environment: There's Nothing New

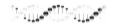

The human part of us asks questions such as "What is going on?" "Why didn't somebody tell me before that I was killing myself with each donut and diet soda?" I know they said I'd get fat, but no one ever said anything about contracting diseases like cancer!

The truth is if it falls inside my hula-hoop, it's my responsibility. The hula-hoop only has room for one, but I have full control and responsibility for everything inside its boundaries. Even if a friend calls and says they want to go shopping, so I go with her and my wallet gets stolen from my purse while we are walking. I can't blame it on her because it was my choice to go with her. to take the right precautions to cover myself. Understand?

So, I am responsible for my hula hoop, and you get to do the same – making decisions that are the best for you in every way. Don't let the opinions of others change the decisions for your health and well-being that you are making. The Father says "Wait, slow down" especially when you're not sure of the next right step. Keep doing the next right thing, and wait for the next door to open. I've found it is much safer that way.

Also, it's amazing how everybody in the house is now willing to eat what mom is cooking, even if it's healthy! They are learning good, healthy life skills that will give them a longer, healthier life. They are learning to choose the right foods and to eat less junk food, which is the secret to preventing disease root. Children who learn a clean and natural way of eating at a young age will be positively changed for the rest of their lives. When the cycle of unhealthy eating is broken, the family can enjoy better health for generations to follow.

> "The enemy comes only to kill, steal, and destroy, but I came that you might have Life and Life more abundantly." Jesus,
> John 10:10.

"When you know better, you do better." Maya Angelou

Cancer is the enemy of the healthy. The only way to overtake an enemy is to fight it with all the ammunition in your arsenal, and fight to win! Cancer is sneaky and evil, and it comes into your body one deformed cell at a time, catching you completely unaware. What you must do, as soon as it is discovered, is attack FULL FORCE!

As far as research can tell, cancer enters your system by what you are consuming, the environment you live in, and in a small percentage of people, the genetics of their family. I'm sure you've heard the old saying, "Keep your friends close, but keep your enemies closer." The plan of attack in this book is directed to identify the monster and bring him down.

Webster's dictionary defines an enemy as one who is "antagonistic to another, one seeking to injure, overthrow or confound; something harmful or deadly; a hostile unit or force." Doesn't that sound like the definition of cancer and what the malformation of cells are trying to do to you?

Life throws curves when we least expect it, but we don't have to let them take us down. I wrote this handbook for you to use to eradicate all cancer in your body, rebuild your system, and most importantly, to prevent diseases from ever invading your life again. I'm convinced that we don't need to use the extremely difficult jargon the medical profession uses. It's obviously not working for them. I share my experience, strength, and hope, so everyone can understand and may come to terms with the disease destroying their own lives.

Statistics on cancer and deaths related to cancer, in the U.S. are staggering. One in four Americans will die from cancer every year, while millions more are diagnosed. Cancer is the second highest killer, exceeded only by heart disease and stroke, according to the American Medical Association. The statistics from the American Cancer Society in 2008 show 23% of the people who get cancer of any type, do not survive. Statistics report that 1 in 9 women will be diagnosed with breast cancer in their lifetime and one in three will die from the breast cancer. (Within the year of 2008, while I was recovering, the number jumped to 1 in 8 women diagnosed!) How can a modern, technological society such as ours stand by and accept these statistics? They may be facts, but they're not the Truth. God has that!

Some History About Cancer

About 150 years ago, cancer was rarely seen in our culture, very rarely diagnosed. About 100 years ago, cancer cells were rarely being detected, but the medical profession began using chemo, radiation, and surgery to treat all types of cancer. Today, in 2017, these three approaches are still the traditional treatments sanctified by the AMA for anyone diagnosed with cancer. Does that sound logical to you?

Technology has progressed exponentially in the past century, so why hasn't the treatments of this deadly disease? In fact, the reported number of deaths from heart disease, combined with the number from cancer, find that one in two people diagnosed here in America will die from the diseases, right here in "The land of the free and the home of the brave!" Statistics like these should be causing authorities alarm.

Rest assured, global statistics in other civilized countries are not much better than ours, but there are some differences occurring because of geography and culture. It would profit America to glean from these societies and utilize some of their ancient secrets.

Take, for instance, the Mediterranean culture. Their diet consists mainly of fruits, vegetables, and freshly-caught ocean fish. EVOO, extra virgin olive oil, a healthy fat, is the only fat used. As a result, their lifestyle reflects a much healthier culture, so therefore, they have a lower death rate from cancer and heart disease. If the U.S. would learn from the Mediterranean culture, we could save thousands of lives by promoting fresh, nutritious foods instead of junk food and fast foods.

I pose this question: Are we going to allow cancer, any type of cancer, to continue to escalate to higher proportions in our society before agreeing to make some significant changes in our prevention and treatment processes? How can we afford to with a death rate like we currently have?

We cannot rely on the same procedures that were used a 100 years ago with pharmaceuticals that are designed only to prolong a diseased life, instead of using acceptable treatments to attack the root of the diseases. These methods have only profited doctors, surgeons, and insurance companies with billions of dollars while leaving the U.S. citizens to suffer. The medical arena operates from the disease concept, which is to put a Band-Aid on it, but American people deserve better than that. There are many alternatives, both mild and aggressive, that could be introduced and put into widespread use in the fight against cancer, but the medical community will not allow them to come out of the labs, and the insurance companies will not add them to their policies.

I am taking the opportunity, and the miracle of my own healing, to prove to women (and men) of all ages that there are better answers. Answers that bring success, but aren't acknowledged by the medical field. I personally showed two doctors, two surgeons, and one oncologist the original and final results of my x-rays, and I explained to them my method for overcoming the cancer and the path I took. Their response was to reason away all the evidence in front of them. They said that it was just a coincidence that would never happen again, but they've come to me too late with this excuse. I have seen recovery happen first-hand, and I'm ready to see it happen in millions more!

It's not going to be easy to open their minds because, in medical universities, they were taught only disease and the Band-Aid concept. Most are not willing to relearn, even at the cost of saving lives, because the medical insurance conglomerate runs the health system in the U.S. Livelihood of the medical profession is supported by the process that is now set up, and diverting from the mainstream means fewer profits for both the medical community and the insurance companies.

I have found only one female gynecologist, an MD, in my medical experiences who has been educated in medical, nutritional, and bio-identical hormones as healing techniques. But we can't all be her patients! More private doctors should take on the challenge of learning nutrition and alternative methods. Her expansive knowledge allows her to implement more choices in her patients' treatments, and she is constantly learning new avenues of healing. Her patients find control over their own bodies, utilizing the type of treatment best suited for their lifestyles.

Whether you have been diagnosed with breast cancer or not, the information in this book will make a tremendous difference in your life by showing you how to make healthier choices. The medical community should be informing the public with updated information on health and healing for their bodies, but any new alternative information from the mainstream, including preventative information, is scarce.

Body, Soul and Spirit

Cancer is a disease that affects the mind, body, and spirit, so all three areas need to be addressed in the recovery process or the chances of retaining the healing is slim. An example of this would be a woman who is diagnosed with breast cancer, so her doctors gave her a mastectomy. They declare that they got all cancer, but in less than a year the same woman is seen again with cancer in the other breast, so surgeons remove that too.

Five years go by, and now her physician has diagnosed colon cancer. She was not treated completely—mind, body, and spirit—from the first incident or the same cancer cells would not have metastasized around her body. There is no difference in cancer cells, it is only the location in the body that determines a different name, such as liver cancer, lung cancer, breast cancer, colon cancer, except for types like leukemia, Lymphoma, non-Hodgkins or Melanoma.

There is an ancient wise saying that says, "Without knowledge - people will perish." If that is true, our population is in big trouble because our hospitals are simply not advancing with the technology available. Our health policies in America leave us wanting, and as a result, people are perishing at an alarming rate.

I believe that the knowledge I acquired during this one year overcoming multi-foci breast cancer will help many women and men of all ages live complete and happy lives in the healthiest of lifestyles. With this information, the reader will learn how to make better choices in his/ her lifestyle, as well as for their children. Children learn by example, and what they see their parents do, they will imitate. If you are making more nutritious choices that improves your lives while also fighting this disease, they will learn by what you are doing.

This global report from the IARC, International Agency for Research on Cancer, includes future generations in their research, and they state that "governments, health practitioners, and the general public should take to urgent action. If nations would get into action now, we could prevent one-third of cancers, cure another third, and provide good, palliative care to the remaining third that need it. There are two main causes of cancer — tobacco and lifestyle."

Dr. Paul Kleihues, Director of IARC and co-editor of "The World." I agree 100%.

The Disease and Free Radicals

According to the National Cancer Society, the definition for cancer is this: "Cancer begins with one cell that divides and reproduces abnormally, and then continues to multiply with uncontrolled growth. These malformed cells can break away and travel to other parts of the body, which is referred to as "metastasis."

You must understand that cancer cells are normal in every human being, to some extent. The cells that have been damaged or deformed in some way in the natural process of regeneration are typically cast out of a healthy body, never causing tumors or problems.

Another culprit in causing malformed cells are random free radical cells that attack healthy cells in their journey around the body. Radical cells are made from the toxins in our food or from poisons in the environment, which attack cell, so in cell multiplication, deformed cells are produced. These toxic, free radicals, bouncing around in your body are trying to attach onto weaker cells that they find, and then they reproduce the deformity into a new cell, and they multiply the deformed cell to form cancerous cells. As the deformed cells are produced, they accumulate and form lumps and tumors, chronic inflammation and bacteria. This is how sickness and cancer enter the body.

Free radical is a relatively new term, but the name fits the cell's personality perfectly. Free radicals are radical cells that have been formed from foreign substances: a chemical spray in the atmosphere or a toxin in the food. They roam freely throughout the body causing destruction. Realistically, it would be impossible to completely protect yourself from all of these invaders, unless you lived in a bubble. The 21st century is extravagantly different from the early 1800s in terms of pollutants.

Free radicals are created by the chemicals in processed food, and the pollution and chemicals in our air; they even come from the chemicals in some cleaning products! If you are lucky enough to live high up in the mountains where the air is pure, even then, you would still be exposed to chemicals created by the microwave, impure water, and water packaged in plastic bottles that have been sitting in hot warehouses.

Environmentally, America is far from what it was 200 years ago when the fields and lakes were fresh and pristine, and cancer was almost non-existent. Nowadays, the U.S. imports more food than we grow, so the public never knows what or how much chemicals were used in the growing and shipping of produce to America. As a word of precaution, make sure to wash all produce very carefully before eating!

Every healthy human being is carrying approximately 2,500 to 100,000 malformed cells on any given day and isn't even aware of it. A human body is made up of trillions of cells, and it takes millions of cells to create a mass the size of a nickel. When the immune system is not as strong and vibrant as it should be, it does not capture the radical malformed cells and dispose of them as effectively as it should. Maintaining a healthy immune system is a top priority.

When your system is healthy and your immune system is strong, you'll have no problems eliminating the few thousand malformed cells your body randomly creates.

A healthy immune system will dispose of them efficiently. The most important fact besides cutting out sugar is to drink fresh clean filtered water throughout the day, so you are continually flushing out the malformed cells.

A normal person, with a healthy immune system, is probably not reading this book, so consider your immune system as one that needs to be strengthened. If you have been diagnosed with a major disease like rheumatoid arthritis, Fibromyalgia, Lupus or cancer, you get colds easily or you have a low energy level, your immune system is compromised. Rebuilding it should be your primary goal in gaining your health back during this next season of your life. With a compromised immune system, your body's defense system is damaged and dysfunctional. By focusing on building it to its prime, you will regain your health and wellbeing. The outline in this book is exactly what you need.

Preventative Care

When practicing a preventative diet and lifestyle, use the medical profession whenever possible to evaluate any inconsistencies you might find because the faster they are found, the sooner you can take care of them. Early detection tools such as mammograms, CT scans, X-rays, ultrasound, and colonoscopies are extremely helpful, but they are not perfect. Recent reports show that about 10% of new breast cancers originate from the radiation emanating from the mammogram machines. Early detection tools need to be developed using advanced technology, so they are more helpful. Be cautious of the equipment your medical facility uses, and don't think twice about doing your homework and questioning your doctor.

Medical Treatments vs. Natural Treatments

It is important to know that once a healthy cell has become malformed, it can never be transformed back into a healthy cell. It must be broken down by the liver and flushed out of the body, and this is the action your body will automatically take. Cancer and cancerous tumors begin with a small number of malformed cells that begin multiplying at breakneck speed when toxic materials and foods enter into the system.

Surgery, radiation, and chemo are used exclusively in the medical community for patients diagnosed with cancer, but these radiation and chemo treatments are anything but true "cures." Radiation consists of microwaves that penetrate the body and attempt to kill the bad cells off. The only problem is that it also kills off just as many good cells and causes massive amounts of deterioration in the body's tissues.

Recent studies show there is NO guarantee for positive results using radiation, and it is the same with chemotherapy. Chemotherapy uses harsh chemicals injected into the body to kill the cancer cells. The way chemo works is that it kills everything in the entire system, whether it is the malformed cells or your own healthy ones, and then attempts to allow the body to replenish itself. Certain kinds of chemo have been known to create other diseases in the body as side effects that also become chronic. It destroys all the good vitamins and enzymes in your system, so if you choose this method, it is imperative that you support your system with vitamins and supplements to help restore the damage. You can improve the recovery from chemo and radiation with the program in this book, altered for your specific needs, and shorten your recovery time immensely.

The other medically-approved procedure is surgery, and in some cases only a small cyst or tumor needs to be removed. But, keep in mind, there is always a risk involved with any surgery, but the removal of a tumor is a relatively safe option. In my case, the surgeon said that a double mastectomy was the only answer, but my left breast was perfectly healthy! All the cancer was in the right. He explained it was "in case the cancer would spread." I'd say he was getting overly happy with the knife, and the expectation of more money.

By the Grace of God, he was proven wrong in six months! I can't guarantee a timetable for everyone because everyone's system is unique, but this book consists of everything that I did for the year and how I changed my life. You only have to change everything, so don't worry. The information in this program is scientifically supported by naturopathic medicine, which is the natural way of life and healing, and as a counselor, I have also found it to be supportive in recovering the mind and emotions. This is an entirely better lifestyle you are going to experience.

If you decide to use any of the three traditional treatments, radiation, chemo or surgery, for whatever reason, know that the power of this natural program will add energy, and for many, a shorter recovery period, while preventing more cancerous cells from forming or metastasizing. Recovery of your immune system requires a diet filled with nutrients to create new healthy cells again. This way of life has even changed my taste buds to appreciate healthier foods and has improved my general perspective immensely.

On December 27, 2007, the fight of my life was presented to me. Any of you who have been presented with this challenge know first-hand what goes through your mind: first denial and unbelief; then defense, fear, and anger; then flight and anonymity, and finally, after all of that, your sense of self returns to you. For some, this process takes a relatively short time and for others, it could take years to regain your composition. Everyone is different, so time is irrelevant, but you have to accept and defend your body when it has been invaded by cancer.

Chapter 2

Life in Your Hula Hoop

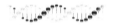

Cancer attacks people of any age nowadays as more processed foods come on the market and the environment has more pollution. Chronic diseases, like cancer and heart disease, used to be expected in the senior years, but today's young children are increasingly being diagnosed with cancer. Unbelievably, this is the first generation that is dying before their parents, which goes against the natural course of life. Parents should pass away first.

When cancer hits someone, it comes without warning. It takes control and becomes an evil foreign force invading your space and body, trying to take over. If you are anything like me, you like to think that as stubborn or complacent as we can be, it is still our right to say what goes on in our personal lives or "everything within our hula-hoop." When that is taken away from us, it's our right to get upset, take action, and fight back. After all, it's our hula-hoop, and it's our life here on this planet.

Hula-hoop? Yes, hula-hoop. Imagine taking a hula-hoop (You remember those, don't you?) and putting it on the floor and stepping into the middle of it. Everything inside that hula-hoop you get to control, with the help of the Creator, of course. When the surgeon told me his diagnosis of breast cancer, my concept of control was shaken to its foundation. I got very angry when cancer tried to take the decision-making ability of my own body away from me. The enemy came into my territory uninvited, but with God on my side, the fight was on.

I understood I was in the center of this hula hoop, and you must, too. For this season of your life, you must let others take care of themselves, so you can concentrate on your diet, your rest time, and your relationship with the Father. You are "numero uno" in your universe until you get the "all clear" report from your final cancer test. It is nothing to feel guilty about; you must put yourself first in order to win this fight. Those close to you will understand and help you all they can, but this is your fight.

So, I began the most horrendous, yet miraculous, year of my life, but by the time I had kicked cancer's butt, everything had turned around 180 degrees. After receiving the shocking report of multifocal breast cancer, I stood up for myself and made total changes for my benefit in my lifestyle, and I now have the best health and spiritual energy I have ever had! There is hope for anyone who reads this book and applies the information they find.

Hope and faith are as tangible as a table and chair after you accept the fact that they are available for you. Receive them now. God already has the solution to fix everything that is broken; He created YOU. You are a self-contained unit created for success. Leave negativity behind, and allow victory to take the place of uncertainty and depression. A challenge is a challenge; take it!

Nothing in my life has been the same since that day in the surgeon's office. Everything has been turned upside down from the norm it was in only two years before. Despite all that, I have found true Peace and Joy deep down inside, and I have discovered how to stay in that peace through the midst of a storm. My life is now on the right path. I'm healed, healthy, and whole, and I'm not going back to a lesser lifestyle. The enemy snuck into my camp with his arsenal of fear, death, and destruction, but I will not have it anymore. I found out that I am strong, and I can fight back! With God, all things are possible.

There is no reason to worry because worry never accomplishes anything. I don't care what the doctor's report was, you have found a safe place here. I have gone through the endless waiting rooms, the uncaring doctors and surgeons, the crying, the isolation, the confusion, the overwhelming feeling that this is way too much for me to handle, and I want you to know that you'll go through it, too. We are all human, but now you have new information and a success story to feed your faith. You'll grow and come back to life as you listen to the next right thing to do. The Creator is in control, and we're going to let Him be all that He is!

The Body, the Cell

The question is, then, "Are we as a culture going to bring any changes to the way cancer is treated, so those afflicted can recover faster and with less destruction?" Granted, a few new medicines have been developed in the past 100 years that are prolonging lives, but this is not a satisfactory answer for the population. If we continue to use the same treatments for cancer that were used 100 years ago, we are not going to find an answer in this century to eliminate cancer. It is unacceptable for us to continue submitting solely to the medical profession without considering other avenues for healing.

There are alternatives that have been used for thousands of years, that if combined with the latest scientific data of today, they only need to be introduced, researched, and accepted as alternative options. Our bodies were meant to heal themselves with the assistance of natural treatments, and many methods have been researched and proven to be successful. But, the AMA and the NCS continue to ignore them.

Super nutrition, herbs, supplements, relaxation, meditation, prayer, acupuncture, and exercise are not too extreme to be incorporated into cancer therapy. They are being used today with great success. A new mindset would change the occurrence of cancer and the way it is treated in the U.S., but more importantly, in your life today. It is unacceptable to continue to rely on centuries-old procedures, using only updated pharmaceuticals to merely mask a disease.

These methods have profited the doctors, surgeons, and insurance companies long enough while leaving patients to suffer. There are many alternatives, both mild and aggressive, which should be introduced to the general public and put into widespread use if we're seriously going to overcome cancer. The AMA and nationwide insurance must acknowledge and accept them for better and more effective treatment.

Human Cells Heal Themselves

As I said before, the human body was designed by God to completely repair itself. You witness this phenomenon whenever you cut your arm. Without any medicine or antibiotics, these minor ailments heal within a matter of days. The body will instinctively call for added fluids and more rest, and the injury is healed. Our bodies are self-contained healing units, and cancer is not any different from any other ailment. By the time you have read this entire book, you'll know just what to do to help your body heal.

This is a struggle for your health that you must fight for yourself, no one else can do it for you. Others can help, but ultimately, it's up to you.

Healthy Cells/ Malformed or Cancerous Cells

There are only two basic types of cells: healthy and malformed, and they are as different as night and day. The healthy cells thrive on nutrients, enzymes, vitamins, fresh, clean water, fresh vegetables, fruits and clean meats. The malformed cells, on the other hand, absorb the "garbage" in the system — including white sugar, white flour, processed foods with long names that nobody can pronounce, chemicals, pharmaceuticals, and the toxins in the environment. These two kinds of cells – the healthy and the malformed are mortal enemies. Which one will live? The one you feed.

Alternate Therapies of Change that Heal Cancer

There are several alternative therapies available that have been researched, tested, and proven. The internet has many success stories about overcoming the enemy of cancer, but of course, they don't fall into the AMA criteria, so you really have to search for them. I will show you natural methods of healing that you can begin to use immediately.

This is not a book to absolutely disclaim the traditional three treatments because you must choose the right solution for yourself, but don't attempt to make decisions without all the information. The alternative methods that I combined for my success could be used with complete confidence as many people have been healed with similar programs or the same treatments could be used with chemo treatments, radiation, and surgery to assist in an intense recovery process. The results would be swifter healing with less pain and fatigue, which are side effects of radiation and chemo.

I had to save myself from the hands of doctors who only knew the words—surgery and mastectomy. I did not agree with them, so I did the only logical thing I could think of, I began to use my college skills of research. I began to investigate what I did not know, and I began to pray. I searched on the internet and talked with a respected Dr. of Naturopath. I have a Master's degree in Sociology, a degree in Ministry and a certificate as a Natural Health Consultant, where I took much of my information after graduating from the Global College of Natural Medicine in San Jose, California. I have spent my life researching and compiling information, and I used that talent to help me immensely as I studied to overcome cancer.

I ask you to read this book with an open mind. You'll receive some things by reading the black letters on the page and applying them to your life, them to your life, while most of the strength and hope you'll receive will come from the white spaces. It's not a complicated process, but it will probably be the most difficult and intense season of your life. Cancer puts up a good fight, but we have the edge. God is on our side! You will have to leave your present lifestyle behind, though, because it obviously wasn't working. Keep your eyes looking forward.

All I can tell you is that if you have found yourself at the point of desperation I reached, seeing no hope and no alternatives, you are about to get a download of hope, grace, and direction that you can use right now. Day by day, you'll begin to pick yourself back up while building your faith. This mountain of illness and disease that overwhelmed you will slowly diminish until you see yourself as the winner, an overcomer. Soon, you'll be walking in the middle of a life so grand and full of possibilities that you won't even recognize it as yours! And you'll never look back because the enemy was defeated!

The rate of cancer has more than doubled from 1920-1970, and from 1970 to now, it has quadrupled or multiplied four times over, yet the AMA continues to research and treat along the same disparaging lines. They are using the same Band-Aid approach as the death rate for cancer rises to contend for first place with heart disease. It is your choice to change your path.

News update: The American Cancer Society estimates that there were 1,685,210 new cancer cases diagnosed in 2016 and 595,690 cancer deaths recorded in the United States alone.

Chapter 3

How Could This Be Happening to ME?

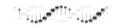

When I'm feeling good and walking on the right path, the Me in me reaches out to help those around me. We are all on this planet and share everything on it, but when I am feeling down or sick, I tend not to reach out, but rather I hibernate and focus on myself. This is not a healthy way to live!

Every person on this planet is unique and should be celebrated, but even as we are so decidedly unique, we are also extremely alike. One obvious similarity is the way our bodies are made, and another is our basic needs. When you consider everything, we are equal, and we share the same emotions and motives. We are generally built the same: two eyes, two arms, two legs and underneath the skin, it's impossible to tell us apart.

The problem arises when thoughts like this run unguarded through our mind - "I can do everything, I am Mom, wife, CEO with three kids; I am superwoman, and I can handle it." With a career, a husband, and kids taking all of our attention, you ask, "When is there any time to take care of myself?" This is the cry of the 21st-century woman, and no one really has an answer for it. Women are achieving more than ever before in the corporate world and are given more choices, but with those choices come more responsibilities, and those responsibilities bring stress.

Stress is a Major Factor in Cancer

Men are feeling the pressure, too. The advancement of women into the once male dominated career place has pushed many a man's masculinities to their limit causing men to compete with women's rising status. Unfortunately, this challenging trend in society has resulted in our bodies retaining more and more stress that never gets released. No one seems to have an answer as to how to release this stress build up, but it has become a tremendous issue in our society today, and stress is a major contributor to the rising cancer rate.

Today, 80% of the population has accumulated stress to dangerously high levels. Science has proven the relationship between accumulated stress and the diagnosis of cancer, so it is important to consider how it is affecting your personal life. Researchers have proven repeatedly that stress is the root cause of all chronic diseases including rheumatoid arthritis, fibromyalgia, Lupus, digestive issues and gut problems along with all types of cancer.

As unique individuals, suffering with a common problem, the answer is in finding a balance for yourself and your unique lifestyle while living in this crazy world. The symptoms of being overstressed manifest differently for each individual, and that's why the world finds it so difficult to diagnose and treat. A place of peace and balance must be found or the stress will take over, with malfunction of every organ in the body. Each person needs to look at his/her circumstances and develop sound habits that allow rest and recovery, instead of chaos, confusion and anxiety.

Stress, in everyday language, affects your body, mind, and soul at the cellular level. Cells that are continually stressed for long periods of time get "stretched" out of shape, similar to the stretching of a rubber band, and the cells are weakened. This means the body must send extra hormones (cortisol) and antioxidants to help combat the situation. Your system then begins to function again, despite the overload, and this becomes a new level that your body gets used to. The next time stress has to be dealt with, more cortisol is sent to help the weakened cells. If this continues to occur, day after day, week after week, year after year, the hormone levels never have a chance to return to normal, and the cell walls never bounce back to their original shape like they were designed to do.

The rest of the world calls this condition "stress," but they do not recognize that it is more than an uncomfortable feeling, and it is destroying their bodies one cell at a time. Scientists show that stress plays such a major role in the disease factor by allowing cells to be weakened and destroyed. No one, doctors or scientists, seem to know how to address the root issue, and millions of dollars are spent each year covering it up with other names to pretend that stress doesn't exist.

Maybe you can relate. You may be having trouble making ends meet. The budget is tight, and stress is building up. You may be caring for a sick family member while raising your own children, managing two households. These are examples of higher levels of stress, and if you're not getting relief, stress builds up and adds more proverbial weight onto your shoulders every day. This pressure is what negatively affects the cells in your body and causes cancer.

As the cell walls lose elasticity and become weaker from being stretched, it is easier for the disease to break in. Your hormone level has now either skyrocketed or plummeted depending on the hormone, and your blood pressure has reached a new high along with your cholesterol level. In this state, there is no peace in your body, so it does not function properly. Of course, there is no peace in your mind and heart when you have reached this state, and your body cannot recover on its own without outside intervention. If you are diagnosed with cancer or another chronic disease, stress adds pressure on the cells, permanently mutating their shape and making them weak, malformed and malnourished, which is our definition of cancer cells.

With added stress, cancer cells multiply rapidly. Can you see why stress and disease are running rampant through the world? This has to be brought to an end. You are now empowered with information on the relationship between cancer and stress, so you can begin to find some calm in your life and respond appropriately to it.

I was always an independent person, until I learned what I was doing to my body. I assumed I was in good health because that's what I wanted to believe. If there is no extreme pain, women especially are programmed from their childhood to maintain a career, home life, and a social calendar, all at the same time. This is expected in today's society, and every woman I know could use more hours in a day!

Children, husband, boss, or friend, someone always needs her time and attention and most of the time, women are more than ready to help. We are nurturers, and we're not very good at saying, "No." Now that you are aware you are aware of this criminal called stress, it's time to "Let it Go!" You are going to have to simplify your schedule and eliminate some of the entries. It's time to start taking care of YOU, so you can create a healthier, more balanced lifestyle.

There is no typical profile of someone "likely" or predisposed to get cancer anymore. With the way our culture eats and the toxic conditions we live in, cancer sneaks into the lives of those who are unprepared and unaware every day. The 21st century has taken us out of control with fast-food diets, too little sleep, long work hours, and no quiet time so that cancer and stress find it easy to invade our lives. Something has got to change and that is us! If you are an average, ordinary, whosoever on planet Earth and you're not taking care of yourself by living a healthy, stress-free or at least stress-manageable lifestyle, then you are left wide open and susceptible to cancer or any other immune deficient disease. If you are already diagnosed, you can recover. This described my life before I learned what I am about to explain to you.

From My Past

Life has not always been a smooth, straight path for me, but up until this point, I have come through all my trials on the learning side. Sometime, many years ago, I heard that every trial is a learning experience, and if I learn something from it, I will be prepared for the next one, especially if the same lesson returns again.

I have been through the usual disappointments life throws at you, missed employment opportunities, disagreements in relationships, automobile accidents, family disputes, and many other unexpected disappointments, but God has never given me more than I could handle with His help.

When I was diagnosed with breast cancer, I thought that God was making up for not giving me any life-threatening situations so far. I thought this might be the last thing I would ever go through. During the process, I discovered that this thought is common among people who are diagnosed with serious, even fatal diseases, but God had a plan for every life, just like He does for yours!

You see, I was adopted at the age of six months, so I never knew my biological parents or genealogical history. This is a huge drawback when you need to know your gene pool origins, such as when you are diagnosed with a major disease. This information would be useful in pointing out weaknesses in your genes, passed down from generation to generation, so your medical history could help explain your condition.

In the 1950s, very little information was exposed when a child was given for adoption. The records were under lock and key up until 1964. The only way for an adopted child or birth mother to get information from a locked file was for both to write a letter of their willingness to share their identity with the adoption agency. The letters were placed inside a file, and if both sides agreed the files would be opened and the identities revealed.

We have come a long way in 60 years! Today, parents are able to adopt children when the biological mother is still pregnant. Needless to say, I never learned who my biological mother and father were or what generational diseases, including cancer, may have run in the family.

But, I often wondered, "How could this be happening to me?" I found out that the disease of cancer can attack anyone who is not actively working a preventative life-style. Simple as that. If you can, check back into your family history. Whether you can find it or not, does not change what you have to do. This program is the answer for complete victory over cancer, and the benefit is great health.

Growing up in the mid-west gave me a wonderful childhood. I have memories of playing outdoors with the other neighborhood kids every day after school, every weekend, and all summer. Video games and cell phones were not invented yet. I had one younger sister who shared my middle-class childhood in Ohio. It was truly an era to cherish.

The world was definitely changed with the explosion of technology. Back then, we were never concerned about being kidnapped or being involved in drive-by shootings in our suburbs because such tragedy hadn't reached that part of America yet. It might have been going on in the larger cities, but it hadn't reached the suburb of Pleasant Ridge.

By the same token, not one of us ever thought about cancer. As far as we were concerned, it didn't exist, but if we happened to hear about someone who had it, it was always about a senior citizen with a depressing prognosis. There was never a thought that we might one day get cancer. We played hard every day until it got dark or we had to go in for dinner. During the late 60s, the Beatles starred on the Ed Sullivan Show and marijuana and other drugs were introduced into society. The Vietnam War was a major topic until they finally started sending soldiers home, and then it was swept under the rug. The drugs changed the American culture, and in the 1970s, the culture began to change in every area.

Coincidentally, the American Cancer Society announced that between 1970 and 1996, the breast-cancer incidence rose from 68,000 cases to 184,300 cases every year. Worlds began to collide. So, I asked myself a dozen more times, "How could this be happening to me?" I was only 49, and I thought I was too young. But, now I was seeing cancer being diagnosed in teenagers and even preschoolers under the age of five. It was happening to anyone.

After I graduated from high school, I spent the next 20 years of my life trying to "find myself." I went to a local college and got a degree in photography, but never did anything with it. In 1996, I went back to college and got a BA degree in Liberal Arts, and then graduated with an MA degree in Applied Sociology. I was a student of the universe. I loved being in school. Since then, I have obtained my certificate in Natural Health Consulting and a license in ministry, which has enhanced my life immeasurably.

From college to the present, I have lived on the east coast of Florida. I fell in love with the ocean, the wind and the waves and have never found it necessary to move back up north. I have to attribute at least a portion of my sense of peace to this environment. The beach and the ocean can take all your troubles away with each wave that washes onshore.

To the Present, Can You Relate?

When I found myself sitting in a surgeons' office waiting for the report from the biopsy, it was a beautiful afternoon as it is so often in December in Central Florida. The months of October through March are truly the reasons why the locals live here. The humidity drops along with the temperature, and all the hurricanes are long gone. What is left are nice, sunny days, with just a hint of coolness in the air. By noon, it usually warms up to a comfortable 75 degrees.

After a short wait, which is surprising for any doctor's visit, the nurse led me back into his office. We'll call the physician, Dr. P. to protect his anonymity. I have known Dr. P. for five years. He also performed my first biopsy In 2004, but on this day, when he and his assistant came into the office, something was different. They both were giving me a "look," with an uncomfortable silence that said, "This is something I don't want to tell you . . . but I have to." I was still trying to think positive. Can you identify with this scenario?

With my first biopsy, they told me the results quickly. It had been a benign calcification, which is fairly routine. I could tell something was different about these results before they even said anything. Finally, Dr. P. spoke sounding so serious. "It doesn't look as good as the last one. I'm sorry to tell you, Ms. Gamble. Your biopsy showed lobular carcinoma, multifocal cancer. I couldn't get it all with the biopsy. I took out the center, but around the whole perimeter, there is carcinoma. I'm afraid what you need is a double mastectomy—nothing less." (Chopping off body parts! What?!)

I was shocked and speechless as the next few moments ticked by . . .

My head was spinning, "They can't be talking about ME! Wait a minute! Let's talk about this! How could this be happening to ME?"

After what seemed like an eternity, which in reality was only a few moments, what came out of my mouth was, "I'm not afraid to die because I know Jesus. If I die, I'll go to heaven—I'm a Christian. My Creator knows me better than I know myself, and He has a much better report than this one. I'm going to get a second opinion." (Since then, I have learned to always get a second opinion on significant diagnoses. Surgeons are quick to want to pull out the knife.)

They both sat there, staring at me with eyes that looked like a deer's caught in headlights. I know you can remember exactly how the news was given to you, too; it was earth-shattering, wasn't it?

I looked over at the assistant, and she started to cry, so I just joined in. I was crying because she was and the shock of it all was so overwhelming, I had to do something! There's no reason to be unnecessarily strong at this moment. Let your emotions and thoughts out. I know if you have already gone through this, you know what I'm saying. It is a tremendous shock, and the reaction is to release those feelings; so, let them go. Don't make any decisions in that state, though. Go home to a familiar environment and make that second opinion appointment.

For about five minutes there was an awkward silence, and the assistant and I just cried because neither of us knew exactly what to say. Then, Dr. P went into automatic mode and started explaining procedures and timetables, giving me other useless information. It was obvious he'd done this a lot, and he began explaining what a mastectomy was actually like, and how with reconstruction no one would be able to tell . . . but, I would be able to tell!

Personally, it was too surreal for him to be confronting me like this. Cutting off body parts is a traumatic message.

He then told his assistant to give me some information about survivor groups in the area while I was asking a few questions about cancer itself. After a few more uncomfortable minutes of awkward questions, I had to get out of that office and away from the hospital, so I could think straight. The office was too depressing. The assistant handed me a few pamphlets, and I quickly left.

Within a few short miles, I found myself on the interstate, headed for home, feeling like someone had kicked me in the stomach. I also knew, though, that I was not going through this alone, that God had made me a born fighter, and this disease was not going to win. I was just barely 50 at the time, which is the new 30, and I was feeling rather comfortable with that. I thought I had been through the hardest days of my life, and that the last half was going to be all downhill. Surprise!

Cancer can happen to anyone! I had to get quiet and give the whole thing to the Father. I went to the beach, one of my favorite places to get quiet and centered. I knew I was in the middle of this battle, but it was not mine; it was God's. He is everywhere and all-powerful, and I am His child. I knew I was going to be required to do the footwork, but the results would be in His hands.

I got home in an hour and went immediately online, looking up breast cancer and how it affects women's bodies. Without knowledge, people perish, so I searched for a surgeon in Orlando for a second opinion. When it was all said and done, throughout the next few weeks, I went to two surgeons, a plastic surgeon, and an oncologist looking for answers.

I went to an oncologist because he was referred by a friend named Michael who had lung cancer, which metastasized along his spine. He was being treated with radiation and chemotherapy. Michael was a wonderful recovery friend who beat this disease by going to a much better place. Michael went to Heaven in Feb 2009, and will always hold a special place in my heart. He was 37, and one of the many reasons I have for hating this disease that has no conscience and no logic. Michael left behind his soulmate and three teenage boys.

All four of the physicians I saw told me the same thing - a double mastectomy was the only answer. Period. Not one of them would keep me in their care without being scheduled for the surgery, either. They all said that according to the AMA and their malpractice insurance, they couldn't cooperate with my choice of using alternative methods because their insurance wouldn't cover it.

I couldn't schedule any more appointments with the surgery they offered, so I cut loose and released myself from medical care. You will find this is one of the hardest things you'll do in recovery, but it is so necessary in order to find another support network that will give more positive and progressive solutions for recovery. The standard treatment of the AMA left me absolutely no control over my own body or any of the treatments related to it.

Does any of this sound familiar? The fear and confusion of getting any positive information was almost overwhelming. I know that the way I was treated is pretty standard. All those diagnosed must start here, where it feels like I was just a number in a sea of patients, and we all were getting the same cold, uncaring treatment. It's cookie-cutter medicine to me. I was one of the hundreds coming through the turnstile into this system that didn't much care about me as a person, and no one was looking for any real answers concerning the cancer I had. The money factor is clearly their priority, so I instinctively knew that if things were going to turn around for me, I was going to have to keep my distance from these stubborn, negative, and one-sighted doctors and enlist in alternative support.

I was trying to stay in peace in the midst of this storm of emotions, and believe me, it was storming, and I had no one to even hand me an umbrella! I didn't have the information that is accumulated in this book; the answers were going to come from areas that I hadn't even found yet, but I knew they were out there, somewhere. God had a plan.

A month went by after I had received the second opinions, and I told each one that I could not participate in the sentence they had subjected me to. It took all the courage I could gather to confront those doctors. The medical system had brainwashed me since birth into believing that they were the exclusive answer to my health. They were gods in their own eyes, but I knew my God, and He did not accept their report. I was to believe the report of the Lord. He sent His Only Son, so I could be healed. Should I turn away from that? It takes more faith to believe in a doctor than to believe God because God is a sure thing!

Another thing is that I didn't feel like giving up or caving in to compromise. The years of my life have always been spent pressing towards a goal, whether school or career. I can easily look back and remember how I've always been learning what life is and applying what I learned.

How is this Really Happening?

Like most females, I have been on a diet of one kind or another my entire life, losing the same 15 pounds over and over again. I thought I knew what healthy and nutritious meant. I thought I was eating just fine, but the truth was that while I was eating lower calories on some days, so I was getting less nutrition.

As I look back, graduate school was a really good time in my life. I was 47 years young, so to all you middle-aged people reading this—47 is the new 27, and now is not the time to be thinking you have nothing left to do in life. God has something spectacular He wants you to accomplish. I have to believe that middle-age is just what it says it is - the middle of our age. We have gathered so much information so far in our lives, and now we're mature enough that God will start letting us use it.

What have you done for the first time since you turned 40? After I graduated in 2004, I taught my first college Sociology class. God did have a plan for my life, and it was funny that I stayed in school this long, only to return to school. This proved the old adage was true that we never really graduate in life. I had become the professional student, and I figured there were many lessons I had learned in school, but there was much more I learned outside the classroom, two of which were perseverance and discipline, and they were yet to come.

The best gift you can receive during this entire situation of being diagnosed with a deadly disease is the Gift of Desperation. You might not realize what that means yet, but if you can hang on for a couple more days, it will fall on you and give you an open mind about everything that crosses your path from now on. The Gift of Desperation lets you release the fears of the unknown and helps you to walk in hope when you don't know any of the answers.

I would like to share some life lessons and inspirational messages from a fellow traveler, Regina Brett, who was diagnosed with breast cancer in 1998. During her chemo and radiation treatments, she wrote these life lessons about her walk. Ms. Brett has a radio show in Cleveland, Ohio, so live and learn.

Lessons in Life by Regina Brett

"To celebrate growing older, I once wrote the 45 lessons life taught me. It has become the most requested column I have ever written. My odometer rolls over to 50 this week, so here's 50 as an update:"

1. Life isn't fair, but it's still good.
2. When in doubt, just take the next small step.
3. Life is too short to waste time hating anyone.
4. Don't take yourself so seriously. No one else does.
5. Pay off your credit cards every month.
6. You don't have to win every argument. Agree to disagree.
7. Cry with someone. It's more healing than crying alone.
8. It's OK to get angry with God. He can take it.
9. Save for retirement starting with your first paycheck.
10. When it comes to chocolate, resistance is futile.
11. Make peace with your past so it won't screw up the present.
12. It's okay to let your children see you cry.
13. Don't compare your life to others'. You have no idea what their journey is.
14. If a relationship has to be a secret, you shouldn't be in it.
15. Everything can change in the blink of an eye. But don't worry; God never blinks.

16. Life is too short for long pity parties. Get busy living, or get busy dying.

17. You can get through anything if you stay put in today.

18. A writer writes. If you want to be a writer, write.

19. It's never too late to have a happy childhood. But the second one is up to you and no one else.

20. When it comes to going after what you love in life, don't take no for an answer.

21. Burn the candles, use the nice sheets, wear the fancy lingerie. Don't save it for a special occasion. Today is special.

22. Over prepare, then go with the flow.

23. Be eccentric now. Don't wait for old age to wear purple.

24. The most important sex organ is the brain.

25. No one is in charge of your happiness except you.

26. Frame every so-called disaster with these words: "In five years, will this matter?"

27 Always choose life.

28. Forgive everyone, everything.

29. What other people think of you is none of your business.

30. Time heals almost everything. Give time, time.

31. However good or bad a situation is, it will change.

32. Your job won't take care of you when you are sick. Your friends will. Stay in touch.

33. Believe in miracles.

34. God loves you because of who God is, not because of anything you did or didn't do.
35. Whatever doesn't kill you really does make you stronger.
36. Growing old beats the alternative—dying young.
37. Your children get only one childhood. Make it memorable.
38. Read the Psalms. They cover every human emotion.
39. Get outside every day. Miracles are waiting everywhere.
40. If we all threw our problems in a pile and saw everyone else's, we'd grab ours back.
41. Don't audit life. Show up and make the most of it now.
42. Get rid of anything that isn't useful, beautiful, or joyful.
43. All that truly matters, in the end, is that you loved.
44. Envy is a waste of time. You already have all you need.
45. The best is yet to come.
46. No matter how you feel, get up, dress up, and show up.
47. Take a deep breath. It calms the mind.
48. If you don't ask, you don't get.
49. Yield.
50. Life isn't tied with a bow, but it's still a gift.

Put your favorite ones on the refrigerator, in the car or anywhere you need a boost and a positive thought. Enjoy one day at a time, keep things simple and remember to breathe. If you can succeed in these few things, you have overcome the thoughts of someone with a life-threatening disease. You are going to succeed!

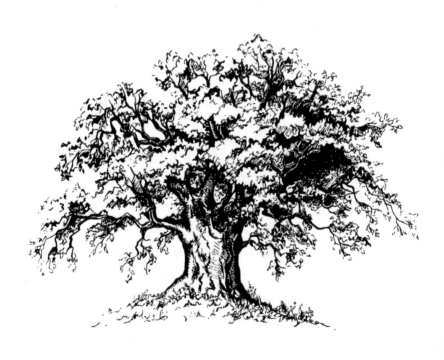

Chapter 4

Breathe, Moments of Reflection

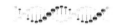

P neuma is the Greek word for breath, wind or spirit. Breathe is what you need to remember to do if you are in this fight for the long haul. The fight you are literally fighting from the inside, out.

Ruwach is the Hebrew word for breath, wind or spirit. Breathe is what you need to remember to do if you are in this fight for the long haul. The fight you are literally fighting from the inside, out.

I am writing this for those who know how to pray and for those who don't because it is essential to recovery. Let this book be a connection, whoever you are. Let it be a connection to life and life more abundantly. I pray everyone who picks up this book and reads it will be changed - physically, mentally and spiritually; and healed completely from the disease you are fighting.

God is Love.

Read with an open mind because you'll only receive some things by reading between the lines.

It's not complicated, it is simple.........but it is not always easy. It is directed and guided.

But, you are not alone. Look inward. There's more than you ever thought.

If you are here with no hope, refresh yourself now. You have found a safe place. The words on these pages are meant for you and your recovery. So relax and find calm and peace. It is going to be OK.

So Pneuma. Breathe Deeply

I have gone through the doctors, the waiting rooms. I know the tears, felt the loneliness and desperation and the overwhelming feeling that this is way too much for me to handle. I want you to know that you'll go through it all too. But not without new information to feed your faith.

Slowly, so slowly that you don't even realize it, you'll grow healthier and come back to life in your soul as you see for yourself what the Creator can do. Chances are that this twist in the road, which has overwhelmed you and has left you with confusion and exhaustion will slowly begin to straighten out until once again. You'll see yourself right in the middle of a life so grand and full of possibilities that you won't even recognize it.

And you'll never look back. So Ruwach. Breathe in and breathe out.

Changing your life is God's way of saying. "You're moving ahead." The habits and routines that you were used to doing obviously weren't working, so it's time to change. If you have been diagnosed with cancer, you are going to change bad habits into good ones that you can use the rest of your life. And it could very well open your eyes to the style of life you are leading right now, completely unaware like I was.

Take this time in your life. Search for Peace, not how to juggle the chaos. There will always be chaos, out there, but we have to live in Peace.

I went from the diagnosis of breast cancer to a clear mammogram in six months, and then exactly one year later, I had a clear MRI to prove it. But the crazy chaos had to be stopped first, so the healing could take place.

Time has no relevance any longer. God does not live in time – He made it only for mankind to live in. The process I learned during this year that I took off from the world and the habits I had changed, literally saved my life. Then, without me seeing it, somewhere along the way, my lifestyle changed. I am not the same person, either inside or out, and I have only God and His Grace to thank for the remodeling. The very same can happen for you!

So Breathe, and again Breathe. There is plenty of Zoë (Life) still left in you. Pneuma.

It is not necessary for you to believe in God right now – it is not the destination, but the journey that produces healing. Healing is a process. This breath will fill you. This breath will bring new life.

This has been the most difficult year of my life, but also the most rewarding. It changed me from the inside, and let me know that it's not all about me. Then, also, this year showed me the most loving, caring Person who loved me first.

So Breathe in the new and Breathe out that old stale air you've been carrying around.

I would not change a moment or the added benefit of losing 16 ugly lbs., lowering my blood pressure and cholesterol levels, gaining my sense of peace and general health or the renewed desire to help others like never before.

I turned it all over to Him because He truly cares, every moment and every single cell at a time. But, if you don't yet believe, don't quit until the miracle happens. This is a story about your success and change as well as mine, so Breathe in deeply, and Breathe out again.

Now pick it up and run with it, gaining strength every step you take. We will confront and tackle this disease together. And you will succeed!

………seeing He gives to all, life and breath
and all things. Acts 17:25

Chapter 5

The Daily Process –
You are What You Eat!

I know you are eager to get started on your nutritious, life-giving path, so in this chapter, I will explain all the details about what to eat and what to avoid. It is an extremely important step in your wellness because most of the different cancers originate either in toxic foods or the toxic environment that you have been exposed to. This chapter consists of the complete map of the process that returns you to health by suffocating the cancer cells.

This is also a complete program to strengthen the immune system and build stronger cells. Most of us were living a lifestyle where we didn't really care what we ate; if it tasted good, we ate it. Now, I am introducing a lifestyle where natural health and convenience combine to create a new way of thinking about the food that you are putting into your body; and I have compiled it all into this one book. Everything you need is at your fingertips, so you can review or expand on any area you want. This is the book I wish had been available to me when I was diagnosed. The breathing and listening exercises, along with the other readings, can easily be incorporated into your everyday life. Trust me, this new way of eating will improve your daily eating habits, so you won't be hurting your body anymore. And the energy you'll get will amaze you!

TruthAboutCancer.com is a good place to start researching cancer, any type of cancer and natural alternatives related to it. Every day you will find access to a number of videos or the latest written studies. You can research superfoods and add recipes to your everyday meals, and there are many testimonies on using natural methods to fight cancer! TTAC was not on the internet when I was fighting; they have emerged in the last few years families had cancer and died. The son began to investigate natural remedies and diets and his whole program expanded into a worldwide outreach. The materials you find there will keep you in a positive state of mind and will empower you with ideas you can use for your own recovery.

Science is always discovering more, especially in the area of natural treatments and remedies because the field is endless. GMO, non-GMO, organic, essential oils and acupuncture are all some of the most recent discoveries being used by many people. The successful results that have come about in the fight against cancer are incredible! Investigate the entire website as well as using this book. I agree with their information 100%.

Like I said earlier, even if you are using surgery, radiation, or chemo your recovery will still be greatly increased by the alkaline diet, exercise, and meditations outlined in this book. The techniques in this book are designed to assist in the recovery of cancer or making traditional treatments more tolerable. This way of life, interpreted in different ways, has been proven to lead to the highest level of health and wellness and to assist in reducing the amount of destruction at the cellular level and tissue that you will encounter in traditional treatments.

If you find good information on other sites and verify it with a knowledgeable source, use it in your fight. You are worth the best treatment you can find. Use this book as a reference and to keep you on the right cancer-fighting path. I have included what is necessary to change your body into one that rejects disease and strives for the best health. The more ammunition against the enemy, cancer, the better.

During my recovery, I could not find one single book or website for the average person like myself to use and find this significant and natural information to fight cancer. I wanted to be healed completely, without a recurrence or another chronic disease developing, and ultimately, I desired excellent health.

I wanted to find a healthy path that was not too diffi-cult or too expensive, so I did the research and the Father had me put this manual together with high-quality, func-tional information that anyone could use and benefit from. I discovered that I could get optimum health and find an alternative, healthy options that used no chem-icals whatsoever. Remember, cancer loves to grow by eating the chemicals and preservatives in your body.

Acupuncture was one alternative that I didn't like. Try it, if you're interested, but be sure to use a reputable acupuncturist. The information in this book is enough for you to overcome any cancer, but conducting further research may give you a wider perspective on certain foods, meditations, remedies, and other treatments.

Most importantly, I want you to share with others how you are taking control of your health and recovery by changing your habits. Your life is created by your daily habits. If they are good, prosperous habits, you will be prosperous, but if they are inconsistent or lazy habits, your attempts will not succeed. This spiritual and nutri-tional lifestyle is intended to treat cancer, prevent other chronic diseases and become a springboard for a dis-ease-free lifestyle. Friends and family will be interested in what you have learned here that is improving the mind, body, soul, and spirit. In other words, this program is recommended for everyone!

This chapter, however, is really for you. This recovery plan is designed to assist you every day in every detail.

Everybody is unique, though, so improvement and success will happen at different rates, and your body will react uniquely to the procedures. God loves everyone and He is no respecter of persons, so I am confident He will be with you, as He is with me in finding the absolute best life possible.

Below are the elements that make up the nutritional part of the program. Use this manual to consistently consult in your fight against cancer. Read it over and over.

Fighting the Disease

Remember and review the other chapters because they'll keep your mind positively occupied and not focused on death and dying, but on moving forward. Incorporate the exercises into your daily schedule, and make fighting the disease your priority right now. MAP it out: M for Meditation, A for Affirmation, and P for Prayer. Include breathing exercises, quiet time, Scripture reading, and brisk walking as a part of your daily routine. Even work takes second place to your recovery needs. Clean out your cupboards of the toxic foods and shop for fresh, whole foods. The process will be simple, but you must be diligent and determined. It will also be fun and very rewarding, so don't give up.

Toxic Foods

Toxic food actually damages body tissue and cells that were healthy, and they also feed the malformed cells. Toxic foods include all types of sugars including white and brown, molasses, maple syrup, white and wheat flour, all artificial sweeteners, such as aspartame and sucralose, all chemicals, pesticides, and steroids that are either added to a food or used in processing. Keep your eyes open for high fructose corn syrup on the labels of sweetened foods and drinks because the industry likes to slip it in. Do not consume anything with this highly processed additive. Reading the labels will become second nature to you in a short time. This is a complete list and I know you don't think there is anything at all worth eating anymore, but just wait. God is going to change your taste buds, and you will come to enjoy the clean, natural foods.

The foods you choose to eat are the most effective way to starve the malformed cells or cancer and to strengthen your good cells. Cancer can't multiply if you're not feeding it, and it wants everything on the toxic list. Malformed cells or cancer cells actually separate these from the other ingredients and feed on them. The less you consume, the faster your fight will be over!

Good In . . . Good Out beats Garbage In . . . Garbage Out.

A Body Cleanse to Flush Out Cancer Cells

A body cleanse became important in my battle, once I learned its purpose and how to use it effectively. The "garbage" or cancer cells must die if you follow the regimen of this book, and that's the purpose of everything you are doing. The body must allow good cells to reproduce, but it also must cleanse away the dead or malformed cells, so healthy cells can take their place.

The best way to do this is with an herbal body cleanse that cleans through your organs, including your colon and liver, because these two, along with the kidneys are the organs that are processing the cancer cells and kicking them out. Toxins are also collected from the system where they are being prepared to be eliminated. They have been accumulating since the day you started eating, so if you have any form of cancer, your body has not been properly handling the deformed cells you have had in your system. An adequately functioning system flushes out those cells daily.

Foods that contain fiber is how your body cleanses itself, but there is not enough fiber in a diet filled with fast foods, junk food, or dead food. The toxic materials in the list are not digested, rather, they are stored in your fat cells, colon, and liver, and they need to be flushed out. The body wasn't designed to store harmful toxins, so it can't digest them, and they build up. Humans were meant to eat pure, whole foods without preservatives, to live in pollution-free air, and to drink pure, clean water. A total body cleanse performed on purpose is one way to flush out toxins. Unless you have one in mind, the 'Smart Body Cleanse' is a national brand that cleans the entire body without fasting in 30 days. The capsules are taken daily along with regular meals.

When you finish the first month, wait three months and do another one. The Smart Body Cleanse can be found at your neighborhood health food store or online for a very reasonable price. I prefer this brand, but of course, there are others that are comparable. Make sure that the cleanse you choose is all-natural and herbal, with no added chemicals, for the best results.

The Wonderful World of Water: Three Types

Water is too often taken for granted, but it is the cleansing and life-giving agent in your fight against cancer. You need to drink as much as you can on any given day. At least 10, 8-ounce glasses is a good guideline. You have probably heard this before, but it is so much more important now, in this season, because you are literally washing dead cancer cells out of your body. However, not all water is created equal!

With your new diet for starving cancer cells and feeding healthy ones, the malformed cells are breaking apart and dying at a much faster rate than if you were not on this program. Everything that goes through the body must be quickly flushed out through the liver and kidneys so that they do not become toxic and hazardous to the body. The same is true of the damaged and dead cancer cells; if they can be flushed out quickly, they will not harm the tissue and organs.

Your body is working 24 hours a day, 7 days a week to clean the toxins out and to heal the destruction they've caused. The pure, clean water you drink flushes out these dead and damaged cells and because you have taken away the sugar, preservatives, and chemicals that they were feeding on, they will die — they must die. Changing your taste buds to prefer whole foods with fresh tastes is the answer. Your system knows that these alien cells are trying to multiply, so it works overtime to rid them from your body. What an amazing system our Creator designed for us!

There is a tremendous difference in water, so if possible, choose the best for your situation. Let's take a quick look at the three types: filtered, bottled, and tap.

1) The absolute purest and cleanest water for your body is filtered water. There are several different kinds of filters, and it would be optimal to have it running through your central water source in your home, so you could use purified water for all your water needs. A reverse osmosis filter, however, installed to your kitchen faucet will provide you and your family with the clean, filtered

water for most of your needs including drinking, making ice, and cooking.

You'll be amazed at how much water you use in a day! The human body is made up of 60% water, so clean water is vital, and acquiring a filter is an investment. When water is filtered, it immeasurably reduces the contaminants entering your body, which decreases available food for cancer cells. The company that installs the filter will provide a list of the toxins and contaminants that their filters out each specific system. They are not all alike, so carefully consider which filter provides the best results.

If you need to justify the money you are spending, imagine drinking those impurities! Adding the reverse osmosis filter must be professionally installed, so when they come to your home, ask if they have a shower model that can be easily added. If not, home stores carry acceptable shower filters. When shopping, you will see other filtering alternatives: filters that manually attach to your faucet for under $75 and water pitchers with replaceable filters for under $30. Typically, you get what you pay for.

2) Bottled water has its pros and cons. It is convenient, but not all brands use a high-quality filtering system, so stick with the ones that have been quality tested such as Aquafina, Smart Water, and Waiakea Hawaiian Volcanic Water. Waiakea also absorbs natural trace minerals as it flows through a volcano in Hawaii. Waiakea is a superior brand, so it would be the first choice. Bottled water by

the case would be extremely expensive and inconvenient to use for months at a time, but it is healthier than tap water, so google a good brand.

Bottled water has another drawback. The plastic bottles of water are stored in hot warehouses for extended periods of time. During this time, the properties of the plastic can seep into the water, which would not be beneficial to ingest. Keep this in mind when choosing your main source of water.

3) Tap water is the last choice while you are fighting cancer. Typically, city water is minimally filtered and filled with impurities including pharmaceuticals and fluoride. Tap water must be filtered in order to prevent the contaminants from entering your body, which is now focused on fighting chronic illness.

Chapter 6

A Typical Day in Your
Wonderful New Life

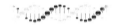

Aim for an Alkaline System

There cannot be enough said about keeping your system at a ph level of 7.4 – 7.8 to keep it alkaline. Science has proven that diseased cells cannot multiply in an alkaline environment, but most Americans would register acidic if tested today. An example of what alkaline means would be if you wanted to grow a plant. It cannot grow in oil; a plant must have water and dirt to grow. To understand this, imagine that thick oil is your alkaline blood system and the water and dirt represent an acidic blood system.

If you place the plant in a pot of oil, it will not grow. It dies. Cancer cells, flu cells, anything that carries disease or bacteria must be in an acidic system to grow because the alkaline system kills it! If you keep the ph level at 7.4, your body will act like a pot of oil and suffocate the plant or disease. This is an extremely effective way in prohibiting diseases and reducing the multiplication of malformed cells. It is easily accomplished by eating the foods from the "alkaline-producing" side of the chart included in this chapter.

The pH scale

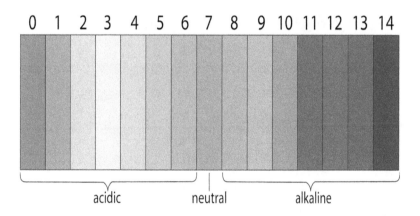

This is a chart of the ph values from acidic to alkaline. You want to aim for the center, 7-8, so you must eat more alkaline foods because any medicines you are taking, acidic foods and the individual chemistries of the human body tend to be more acidic.

How to Measure Your Ph Levels

Keeping track of your ph level is a significant way to boost recovery, and it is very doable. Saliva measures your ph with litmus strips, right at home. The litmus strips can be found at health food stores, drug stores or online, and they typically are available in boxes of 100-200 for approximately $6-$16. Litmus paper comes in small two-inch strips that turn different colors to identify varying levels of acidity and alkalinity. If the paper turns red, pink, or purple, it is reading acidic. If the solution reads alkaline, it will turn blue or blue/green. The alkaline level for recovery must stay between 7.4 - 7.6, and the composition of saliva should turn the litmus paper a dark green/blue color.

Saliva is the best indicator because it registers very close to what a blood test would show at your physician's office. A reading below 7.0 indicates acidity and anything above 7.0 will indicate alkaline. There should be a chart with an explanation on the package. The purpose of testing the level of acidity in your body is to alert you as to whether you are eating quality non-acidic foods, so your system will remain alkaline at all times. The fate of your future is here in your ph.

Cancer cells actually excrete acid, which causes the body's ph level to decrease, lowering your alkaline level. Processed foods and sugar lower the ph level, as do any medicines you are taking. If you continually find that your litmus tests show an acidic level, then remove a few of the acidic foods and add more alkaline foods to bring your system to a good ph level. Barley and other greens, such as alfalfa, will add alkaline quickly, and these greens can be purchased in capsule form to help you maintain the ph level 7.2-7.6. The good news is that you won't have to do this forever. As soon as you are cancer-free, you can add more foods into your diet.

After you have purchased your litmus strips, test several times during the day for about a week, and note the difference in the readings when you eat or don't eat certain foods. As you acquire a healthier diet, the tests will not vary as much. Don't worry. You're doing fine.

Human bodies thrive on healthy fruits, vegetables, and lean meats. Clean meat refers to organic, grain-fed meat from animals that have not been subjected to steroids and added processing. Many meat companies, especially chicken manufacturers like Perdue, are now raising clean chicken with no steroids, preservatives or added fluids that plump up the chicken. Always read the packages at the store; FDA requires all ingredients to be listed on the labels.

The chart is divided into two categories. You'll want to aim at selecting at least 80% of your daily diet from the alkaline side and 20% from the acidic side. This should keep your system sufficiently alkaline, but you'll see when you test. While you are fighting, the closer to 100% alkaline foods that you can eat, the better.

When you are cancer-free, you can add more. I wanted to give the malformed cells no room at all, so I chose virtually all my foods from the alkaline side while I was fighting the fight. Cancer cannot live in this environment.

Every disease automatically causes your system to lean towards an acidic reading if no adjustments are made. Medicines or any pharmaceuticals you may be taking will also cause a more acidic system, so compensate by eating more alkaline foods. Simply keep the chart on your refrigerator or in your purse, and when you go shopping, you should have no problems.

Unfortunately, most people wait too long to adopt a healthy lifestyle of nutrition. It typically takes tremendous amounts of pain before most people are willing to make the necessary changes. Don't put this off!

You are now choosing the best path to restructure your system and improve your life. There is no reason to wait until you have a fatal or even serious disease to make positive changes in your diet. Look around you. There is NO reason to fill your body with sugar-laden and processed foods that hold little nutritional value and are poison to your system. These foods produce acidity and bring nothing but pain and eventually death. Changing your habits only means getting and following new information.

Here is the acid/alkaline chart you can use to select alkaline foods.

ALKALINE FOODS

ACID FOODS

VEGETABLES	FRUITS	MEATS	DAIRY PRODUCTS
Artichokes	Avocado	Pork	Milk
Arugula	Coconut	Lamb	Eggs
Asparagus	Grapefruit	Beef	Cheese
Avocado	Lemon	Chicken	Cream
Basil	Lime	Turkey	Yogurt
Beets	Pomegranate	Custaceans	Ice Cream
Broccoli	Rhubarb	Other Seafood (apart	
Brussels Srpouts	Tomato	from occasional oily fish	
Cabbage		such as salmon)	
Cabbage Lettuce			
Capsicum/Pepper	**DRINKS**	**OTHERS**	**DRINKS**
Carrot			
Cauliflower	Almond Milk	Vinegar	Fizzy Drinks
Celery	Fresh Vegetable Juice	White Pasta	Coffee
Chives	Green Drinks	White Bread	Tea
Collard/Spring Greens	Herbal Tea	Wholemeal Bread	Beers
Comfrey	Lemon Water (pure water	Biscuits	Spirits
Coriander	+ fresh lemon or lime)	Soy Sauce	Fruit Juice
Cucumber	Non-sweetened Soy Milk	Tamari	Dairy Smoothies
Endive	Pure Water (distilled,	Condiments (Tomato	Milk
Endive	reverse osmosis, ionized)	Sauce, Mayonnaise etc.)	Traditional Tea
Garlic	Vegetable Broth	Artificial Sweeteners	
Ginger		Honey	
Grasses			
Green Beans			
Kale	**SEEDS, NUTS & GRAINS**	**CONVENIENCE FOODS**	**FATS & OILS**
Kohlrabi			
Lamb's Lettuce	Almonds	Sweets	Saturated Fats
Leeks	Any Sprouted Seed	Chocolate	Hydrogenated Oils
Lettuce	Buckwheat Groats	Microwave Meals	Margarine (worse than
Mustard Greens	Caraway Seeds	Tinned Foods	butter)
New Baby Potatoes	Cumin Seeds	Powdered Soups	Corn Oil
Okra	Fennel Seeds	Instant Meals	Vegetable Oil
Onion	Hemp Seeds	Fast Food	Sunflower Oil
Parsley	Lentils		
Peas	Sesame Seeds		
Pumpkin	Spelt		
Radish			
Red Cabbage			
Red Onion			
Rutabaga			
Spinach			
Sprouts			
Squash			
Turnip			
Watercress			
White Cabbage			
Zucchini			
FATS & OILS	**OTHERS**	**FRUITS**	**SEEDS & NUTS**
Flax	Sprouts (soy, alfalfa,	All fruits, aside from	Peanuts
Hemp	mung bean, wheat, little	those listed in the	Cashew Nuts
Avocado	radish, chickpea,	alkaline column.	Pistachio Nuts
Olive	broccoli, etc.)		
Evening Primrose	Hummus		
Borage	Tahini		
Oil Blends			

General Guidance:

Stick to salads, fresh vegetables and healthy nuts and oils. Try to consume plenty of raw foods and at least 2-3 liters of clean, pure water daily.

General Guidance:

Steer clear of fatty meats, dairy, cheese, sweets, chocolates, alcohol and tobacco. Packaged foods are often full of hidden offenders and microwaved meals are full of sugars and salts. Over cooking also removes all of the nutrition from a meal.

Credits to Phmiracle.com

Questions

I know what your next thoughts are: "What, why and when are the best foods for me to eat then?" Don't worry. Delicious meals will become second nature to you in time. You can mix and match all the alkaline foods, and before long, you'll find that many of these amazingly good, anti-cancer foods will become your favorites, and they will fit easily into your new healthy lifestyle.

• What are the best foods for my meals?

Now that you know the difference in the foods you are consuming, let me give you the easy answer. Like I said before, when you are fighting cancer, choose many of your foods on the alkaline side of the chart or 80% alkaline and 20% acidic. It is possible to eat only the foods from the alkaline side, plus protein, such as clean meats or organic whey protein shakes. You may lose weight; I did.

Almost a decade later, I still eat basically the same, but on any given day I might adjust my diet and add other foods such as red beans, corn, sweet potatoes or blue corn chips to add variety to my meals. While you are in the fight, they are not allowed. Cancer cells would like the added sugar too much and would multiply! I definitely treat myself every so often and watch for foods that are not essentially "bad" for you, but they produce sugar when they're digested.

- Why do I eat?

Good, healthy, natural whole food is going to be a delight to your toxic-laden system, and it will be ammunition to strengthen the good cells, which in turn, will eliminate the malformed cells. Nutrient-rich foods are necessary for your body. Now is not the time to fast contrary to some beliefs. You need to keep your body at a high-functioning level of performance to overcome the malformed cells. There will be plenty of time to fast after you are completely healed. For now, though, eat a lot and stockpile ammunition.

- When do I eat?

Literally, eat as much of the good, natural, nutritious foods as you want. Alkaline foods are good fuel to fight with, so five or six smaller meals a day is perfect to keep your blood sugar balanced and your good cells stocked with incredible nutrients.

WARNING! Be vigilant! The amount of coffee you drink, even if it's only one cup, will affect your alkaline level. So, be diligent with your litmus tests.

Here's an Outline for a Typical Day—Adjust to Your Taste, but Don't Stray Far!

Start every day by drinking 8 ounces of filtered water, before you even put your feet on the floor. Place a bottle on the bedside table before you go to sleep at night, and then it's right there when you wake up. If you want to add a teaspoon of lemon juice, that's even better. The glass of water wakes up your system and prepares it for the day. Then, have a cup of tea with honey and do some MAP or Meditation, Affirmations and Prayer to start the day.

Taking your AM supplements is important. I suggest filling a pill container at the beginning of the week with the entire week's pills. This will make it convenient to take them morning and night. Take them with food, so that the acid in your stomach that is used for digestion doesn't destroy the pills before they can be absorbed. If you're not having a meal, toast a slice of Ezekiel 4:7 bread to accompany them.

- Breakfast can consist of eggs, plain or with sautéed veggies in an omelet, over easy on a slice of Ezekiel bread with butter, have a whey protein shake with fruit/berries or some goat milk yogurt with nuts sprinkled on top. These are great ways to start the day! You'll notice that protein is the star of these choices and that is perfect for the first meal of the day. It takes longer to digest a protein than it does vegetables or fruit, so you'll feel satisfied longer and have a steady flow of energy.

- A few hours later, juice a glass of fresh, green juice. The instructions and recipes are given in Chapter 13. You can have juice any time throughout the day, but a fresh-squeezed juice for a mid-morning or afternoon treat is a healthy habit to get into. The abundance of nutrients in a glass of fresh juice will make your good cells very happy!

- Later, have a Romaine salad with mushrooms and sliced zucchini with sunflower seeds on top. Make a light vinaigrette for the dressing and add sliced chicken or a sliced hard-boiled egg to give your salad protein and longer satisfying power. Find the recipes in the last chapter.

- Snack all day on fresh vegetables or a mixture of sunflower seeds, pumpkin seeds, and almonds. Hard-boiled eggs are always a good protein that you can make in advance and keep handy in the refrigerator for a snack all by themselves, a delicious egg salad or a great addition to a salad and sandwich.

- Another great lunch choice is an 8-oz. broiled chicken breast, lean ground beef patty or a piece of wild salmon served with plenty of fresh or frozen veggies. (Take supplements with meals as needed.)

- A snack is definitely fine if you desire. Have a small sandwich on Ezekiel bread, homemade trail mix or mixed vegetables.

- Around 6 or 7 pm, have a protein. You can add the protein to Cabbage Soup (recipe in Chapter 13) or have a ½ sweet baked potato and veggies with it. (no white potatoes, they digest as sugar.)

Take your supplements for the night with a snack of applesauce with blueberries and chopped walnuts, yogurt or a cereal that fits the profile with no preservatives or sugar, and then you are free to relax for your breathing exercises and MAP. Find a good book to read to sleep. There is no reason to watch the news, which only highlights violence and murder, because it replays over and over in your subconscious as you sleep. You'll never get a restful night's sleep. This negativity is not good for a healing mind and spirit to watch or read.

Bread - Good or Bad???

Unfortunately, all flour-based bread, even whole wheat bread, assimilates to sugar when it is digested, so no flour-based bread while fighting cancer. Try Ezekiel 4:9 sprouted bread, up to two to three slices a day; it's delicious! Typically, Ezekiel 4:9 bread is sold in health food stores or in the freezer department of better grocery stores, and there are several varieties including cinnamon-raisin and sesame. Ezekiel 4:9 bread is permitted because it is made with sprouted seeds, and when it is digested, it does not turn to sugar like a flour-carbohydrate does; it digests like a vegetable. Ezekiel 4:9 also makes spaghetti and pasta, and they are acceptable for the same reason as the bread.

After you have been totally healed, I would suggest continuing with the Ezekiel line, but you will be able to eat 100% whole grain and other sprouted breads by then. White, processed bread causes bacteria growth in the body, so you want to stay away from it completely, and this includes rolls and other specialty breads.

What can I Drink?

Sodas and drinks with sugar or artificial sugar are definitely off-limits. This is extremely important for several reasons, but too much sugar or artificial sugar are the main reasons. Sodas are simply empty calories that your body does not need to waste time digesting when it could be fighting, and both will hinder the progress you're making.

The beverage to turn to is tea. There are so many herbal teas that are fantastic for recovery because they have no sugar, and they are filled with flavonoids, which are like miniature natural vitamins found in the tea leaves. There are a large variety of herbal teas to add nutritional value while washing away malformed cells.

Try them either hot or cold. Esiak Tea has been scientifically linked to healing cancer, and it tastes delicious. Green Tea is packed with amazing antioxidants, and all herbal teas have individual healing properties. Every type of tea is beneficial, so mix and match and enjoy a variety of flavors.

Sparkling waters with natural flavors also make a good alternative to soda, and 100% natural fruit juices, in moderation, are tasty thirst-quenchers.

Chapter 7

Good Food is a Good Idea

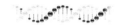

Milk and Other Dairy Products, such as Cheese and Yogurt

While you are in the fight, cow's milk or any dairy products are not suggested, but there are plenty of alternatives that include almond milk, rice milk, goat's milk and if you are a woman, soy milk, in moderation. You can experiment with natural organic cheeses to find the ones you prefer. Organic cheeses have a richer flavor than dairy cheeses, but they are delicious. Make sure the label specifies organic. Meats and dairy products must be organic because of the steroids and chemicals that the animals are injected with as well as the preservatives that are used in processing. Here is an informative article about the relationship of dairy to cancer.

Research Article by Professor Jane Plant on Cow's Milk and Cancer

Below is a short excerpt from "Your Life in Your Hands" by Professor Jane Plant. She recognized that by not using milk or dairy products while fighting cancer, her tumors disappeared. If you get the chance, read the entire book. It is extraordinary. Ms. Plant and her husband were both scientists when she discovered she had five tumors she could feel, and they were measurable. Since they were both scientists, she decided to use scientific research to treat these tumors with no medical interference and closely monitor their results.

Jane and her husband measured the tumors and began to monitor the progress. They researched many different cultures around the globe and noticed that the Chinese have a phenomenally low rate of cancer, which coincided with their low intake of dairy as a nation. Ms. Plant used the information in their research for her recovery. She and her husband found a correlation between dairy products and ovarian cancer in women and prostate cancer in men. This is an excerpt from her book:

"I knew no Chinese people who lived a traditional Chinese life who ever used cow milk or other dairy food to feed their babies. The tradition was to use a wet nurse, but never, ever, dairy products. Culturally, the Chinese find our Western preoccupation with milk and milk products very strange. Milk, I discovered, is one of the most common causes of food allergies. Over 70% of the world's population is unable to digest the milk sugar, lactose, which has led nutritionists to believe that this is the normal condition for adults, not some sort of deficiency. Observing the Chinese diet, I decided to give up not just yogurt, but all dairy products, immediately. Cheese, butter, milk, yogurt and anything else that contained dairy in it.

"I now believe that the link between dairy products and breast cancer is similar to the link between smoking and lung cancer.

"I believe that identifying the link between breast cancer and dairy products and developing a diet specifically targeted at maintaining the health of my breast and hormone system, cured me. It was difficult for me, as it may be for you, to accept that a substance as 'natural' as milk might have such ominous health implications."

Extracted from Your Life in Your Hands, by Professor Jane Plant. In its entirety - http://kanjeex-anytopics. blogspot.com/2007/07/why-i-believe-that-giving-up-milk-is.html

Use the chart below to find foods that will help you combat cancer and add antioxidants to your system. Nuts are good and good for you! Try natural, raw almonds, pistachios, or pecans, which will contribute to your alkalinity and a healthy ph level. Sunflower and pumpkin seeds or Pepitas are delicious to combine, and you can add almonds and raisins to make a homemade trail mix, which is high in alkalinity, good oil, and nutrients.

Tip - Plan the day ahead and keep a bag of homemade trail mix in your purse or car for a quick fix. It is difficult to find healthy, organic snacks when out shopping or at work, so make a big batch ahead of time to last all week. Snacks are unavoidable throughout the day, but find ones that are not sugary and cholesterol-filled, so you don't undermine everything you have been working so hard to accomplish. Choose snacks that support the good cells, so the cancer cells will die out.

Food Chart Listing Nutritional Benefits for Whole Foods

This food chart is the absolute best chart I have seen. At a glance, you can find good foods and see their benefits. Check the chart when you want a snack or to see what nutritional, tasty foods you can add to main dishes.

Apples	protect the heart	improve lung capacity	cushion joints	prevent constipation; block diarrhea
Apricots	fight cancer	control blood pressure	preserve eyesight	shield against Alzheimer's; slow aging process
Artichokes	aid in digestion	lower cholesterol; protect the heart	stabilize blood sugar	protect against liver disease
Avocados	heart healthy	fight against diabetes; help stop strokes	lower cholesterol; control blood pressure	smooth the skin
Bananas	strengthen bones; good source of potassium	control blood pressure; protect the heart	prevent diarrhea	quiet a cough
Beans	help alleviate hemorrhoids	lower cholesterol	combat cancer	stabilize blood sugar
Beets	fight cancer	strengthen bones	aid weight loss	protect the heart

Blueberries	superfood	antioxidant	boost memory	combat cancer
Broccoli	strengthens bones	saves eyesight	combats cancer	controls blood pressure; protects the heart
Cabbage	combats cancer	prevents constipation; helps alleviate hemorrhoids	promotes weight loss	protects the heart
Cantaloupe	saves eyesight	controls blood pressure	lowers cholesterol	combats cancer; supports immune system
Carrots	save eyesight	protect the heart; promote weight loss	combat cancer	prevent constipation
Cauliflower	combats prostate and breast cancer	strengthens bones	banishes bruises	guards against heart disease
Cherries	protect the heart	combat cancer	end insomnia	slow aging process; shield against Alzheimer's
Chestnuts	promote weight loss	lower cholesterol; control blood pressure	combat cancer	protect the heart
Chili Peppers	aid digestion; boost immune system	soothe sore throat	clear sinuses	combat cancer

Figs	promote weight loss	help stop strokes	lower cholesterol; control blood pressure	combat cancer
Fish	protects the heart	boosts memory	combats cancer	supports immune system
Flax	aids digestion; boosts immune system	battles diabetes	protects the heart	improves mental health
Garlic	kills bacteria	fights fungus	lowers cholesterol; controls blood pressure	combats cancer
Grapefruit	protects against heart attacks; helps stop strokes	promotes weight loss	combats prostate cancer	lowers cholesterol
Grapes	save eyesight	conquer kidney stones	combat cancer	enhance blood flow; protect the heart
Green Tea	combats cancer	protects the heart; helps stop strokes	promotes weight loss	kills bacteria
Honey	heals wounds; fights allergies	aids digestion	guards against ulcers	increases energy

Lemons	protect the heart; control blood pressure	combat cancer	smooth the skin	stop scurvy
Limes	protect the heart; control blood pressure	combat cancer	smooth the skin	stop scurvy
Mangoes	boost memory; shield against Alzheimer's	combat cancer	regulate thyroid	aid digestion
Mush-rooms	control blood pressure; lower cholesterol	kill bacteria	combat cancer	strengthens bones
Oats	lower cholesterol; battle diabetes	combat cancer	prevent constipation	smooth the skin
Olive oil	promotes weight loss	protects the heart	combats cancer	smooths the skin
Onions	reduce risk of heart attack	combat cancer	kill bacteria; fight fungus	lower cholesterol
Oranges	support immune system	combat cancer	protect your heart	strengthen respiration
Peaches	aid digestion; help alleviate hemorrhoids	prevent constipation	combat cancer	help stop strokes

Peanuts	protect against heart disease; lower cholesterol	promote weight loss	combat prostate cancer	aggravate diverticulitis
Pineapple	aids digestion; blocks diarrhea	strengthens bones	relieves cold symptoms	dissolves warts
Prunes	slow aging process; boost memory	prevent constipation	lower cholesterol	protect against heart disease
Rice	protects the heart	battles diabetes	conquers kidney stones	combats cancer; helps stop strokes
Strawberries	combat cancer	protect the heart	boost memory	calm stress
Sweet potatoes	save eyesight	elevate mood	combat cancer	strengthen bones
Tomatoes	protect prostate	combat cancer	lower cholesterol	protect the heart
Walnuts	lower cholesterol; protect against heart disease	combat cancer	boost memory	elevate mood
Water	promotes weight loss	combats cancer	conquers kidney stones	smooths the skin
Watermelon	lowers cholesterol; controls blood pressure	protects prostate	promotes weight loss	helps stop strokes
Wheat germ	combats colon cancer; prevents constipation	lowers cholesterol	helps stop strokes	improves digestion

Wheat bran	combats colon cancer; prevents constipation	lowers cholesterol	helps stop strokes	improves digestion
Yogurt	supports immune system; aids digestion	guards against ulcers	strengthens bones	lowers cholesterol

So now, we agree that you want to eliminate white sugar, white flour, chemicals, steroids and processed foods. This includes all fake or artificial sweeteners; they are a slow death. Here is the proof.

The Truth About Aspartame and Artificial Sugars

Walk down any grocery aisle and read some of the labels of the products. You'll find the most popular, processed foods are always located at eye level. Unfortunately, the average American's diet comes from that eye-level shelf, which consists of products with a list of ingredients and words too long to pronounce and white sugar and flour. It is common knowledge that sugar and flour lead to more calories, but the chemical additives produce toxic weight gain. This happens when the body stores the empty foods in your fat and muscle tissues after digesting them. Body cleanses will do their best to clear these out, but you must stop feeding your body unnatural foods that contribute to the buildup.

The problem is that food producers want to make multi-millions of dollars in profits, so they put those toxic foods at eye-level so the buyer can't miss them. Diet brands fill the shelves, but read some of the labels. They are filled with artificial sugars and ingredients, which makes the entire "diet" concept very misleading for consumers. People get addicted to the fake ingredients in these products, and they will spend their food budget picking up quick and easy packaged foods that are filled with poisonous artificial sugars and chemical ingredients instead of eating good, natural whole foods. Keep your list of alkaline and acidic foods with you at all times, so you can make better choices.

Artificial Sugar and Aspartame

Artificial sugar is disguised with names like Aspartame, NutraSweet, Equal or Spoonful, and they are made convenient to the public in the little pink, blue, and yellow packets in every restaurant across the country. This same artificial sugar is exactly what food manufacturers add to sweeten every diet product including drinks and sodas, and they are lethal.

Aspartame was first formulated for the public 60 years ago, and the quality of this chemical has not improved; it is still extremely toxic to the human body. The rule of thumb is that if the label says diet anywhere on it, do NOT eat it. The reason is because it will contain some form of artificial sugar like Aspartame. They could be called Equal or NutraSweet, but they have to be eliminated from your diet. Safe ways to add sweet flavors to foods are with Stevia or honey.

Obviously, the food companies are not going to tell you about the dangers of artificial sugar, but as you can see, it is extremely dangerous to keep using these products. High fructose corn syrup causes inflammation and cancer, but it is another dangerous sweetening agent freely added to foods. Aspartame poisoning and methanol toxicity are very dangerous to the cells in the brain, and the concern comes solely from artificial sweeteners. Alzheimer's is growing in the United States, and the mass misuse of artificial sweeteners is contributing.

Methanol poisoning occurs when the preservatives in lunchmeat or pepperoni, called nitrates, are eaten in a meal accompanied by a diet soda. The nitrates combine with the toxins in the artificial sweetener in the diet soda, and the combination creates a deadly chemical reaction during digestion. Methanol poisoning can lead to death. This may sound far-fetched, but God designed our human bodies very skillfully, and He made them to run on natural foods, not on artificial ones.

Read this astounding information about the digestion of Aspartame. Hopefully, you'll never have a diet soda again.

Our bodies maintain a constant temperature of 98.6 degrees, making us the most efficient heat burner on the planet. We can eat just about anything in the natural world with impunity. The problem is that as soon as chemicals are introduced into the body and the reactions begin, trouble erupts. When Aspartame is ingested, the metabolic breakdown begins. When the temperature of this sweetener exceeds 86 degrees (our temperature is 98.6), the wood alcohol converts to formaldehyde and then to formic acid – which then, in turn, causes metabolic acidosis. Formic acid is the poison found in the sting of fire ants and formaldehyde is the solution used in laboratories to 'pickle' their samples.

Someone who has too much artificial sweetener in their system can find some of the following symptoms alarmingly common: systemic lupus, fibromyalgia-type symptoms, vertigo, dizziness, headaches, tinnitus, joint pain, unexplainable depression, anxiety attacks, slurred speech, blurred vision or memory loss or multiple sclerosis, none of which have proven deadly, but the methanol toxicity is. This is horrendous! What is even scarier is that people contract these symptoms from their diet drinks and sugar-free foods completely oblivious to the cause. Aspartame is causing the symptoms you have taken to your physician, who is totally unaware of the source, so he treats it by the textbook, which means with drugs.

Documented cases show how serious This problem is, but there are ways to combat artificial sweeteners. First, eliminate diet soda entirely. Then, make it a practice to read the labels of food to check for aspartame or other artificial sugars. A good rule of thumb is this: if it says "diet" or "sugar-free" anywhere on the labeling; drop it like a hot potato!

But doesn't that mean you must eliminate all sweets from your diet? No. There is a wonderful, all-natural product called Stevia, which is available in most grocery stores and health food stores. Add Stevia to anything! It is naturally sweet and delicious, so you can have as much as you want - the opposite with aspartame. Promise yourself you'll never use artificial sweeteners again!

Fresh fruits and honey are naturally sweet, but with fructose sugar. If you are fighting cancer, you do not want to have the honey until you are cancer-free, and it is best to keep fruits to a maximum of three servings a day.

All Sugars Are Not Created Equal.

White refined sugar is by far the worst type of sugar for anyone, not just those in the fight. It is the basic product that results when the sugar plant is fully pro-cessed. It has no food value whatsoever, so you are not adding anything beneficial in the way of nutrients when you add sugar. You are only supplying the cancer cells with food to multiply.

The fact is, sugar damages the physical body when you ingest even a tablespoon. It raises the sugar level in the body almost immediately, sending your system on a sugar high. Have you ever given a 5-year-old candy before bedtime? The child can't get to sleep for two or three hours, and this heightened energy blast lasts as long as those sugar crystals are in the blood system. Then the child crashes.

This sugar reaction is the same with adults, but adults have become immune to it after thirty years. The common reaction is to chase the high again. This is so unhealthy for anyone of any age. The body was not meant to have these extreme highs and plunging lows, day after day, because it throws the hormones off balance. Diabetes is a common example of the consequences of this kind of eating where glucose and insulin are not in control of your natural system rhythm any longer.

Brown sugar isn't much better. Many think it is because the color suggests that it's more natural, but brown sugar is simply white refined sugar with added molasses. It is slightly less refined than white, but it still has zero food value and affects the body in the same way.

Fructose is the natural sugar found in fruit and honey, but it is digested completely different than processed sugars. When a food has not been processed, it gets released into the system much more slowly and is easily digested. The sugar highs and lows do not exist. There are many nutrient guides available online, so you can check the grams of fructose in any fruit, but Three to four servings a day of any fruit is a good guideline.

Strawberries and watermelon taste sweeter than Granny Smith apples because there is more fructose in them, but all are fruit. Fruit can be eaten fresh or frozen, whole or diced and added to many recipes. They can be blended in a blender for a smoothie or a food processor to make delicious sauces and more, but avoid canned fruit with added sugar. This will feed the disease. Look for fruit in natural juices. Learn to make all sorts of different dishes with whatever fruit is in season. Be creative!

Adding Supplements and Vitamins

I saved the best and the most important tool in your fight until last. The entire program is designed to work together to form a healthy, disease-kicking lifestyle, but the added vitamins and supplements comprise a major component in your recovery and will have a powerful effect. Supplements are like the exclamation points on your nutritious eating. Up to this point, before you began to fight the disease of cancer, your eating and exercising habits weren't working. The evidence is that you got sick.

Something has to be done to strengthen your defenses. Your body system has to be strengthened from the inside-out, so it can effectively kick out the cancer cells. If you were taking any supplements before, this program is going to go way beyond a daily vitamin or an occasional vitamin C tablet. We are pulling out the heavy artillery because intense measures need to be taken to destroy the malformed cells.

The immune system is called the protector and defender of the rest of the body. It is the system that orchestrates all the other systems when capturing the free radicals that are causing cancer. One of the main reasons for adding the supplements is to support and strengthen that system. The immune system supports the blood system by adding oxygen, and since disease cannot live in oxygen just like it cannot live in an alkaline system, a healthy immune system is extremely valuable.

If you have found a good, well-stocked health food store, take the opportunity to stop in and discuss the supplements you'll need for success. By doing this, you'll take ownership of your recovery and meet a great ally for future questions.

Find out the daily vitamins they stock. A good multi should include vitamin A, B, C, D3, E, K and minerals including manganese, magnesium, calcium, zinc, and others. Make sure zinc is included because it has been found to fight cancer, and it is necessary for good health. Try a liquid vitamin supplement because it is absorbed into the system much easier, and you need to get the nutritional benefits as quickly as possible. Sometimes, when taking capsules or tablets, they do not completely digest, so the full benefits are not obtained. A liquid multi eliminates this problem.

Now it's time to get serious and bring out the heavy artillery. These 14 supplements are essential in attacking the malformed cells. They are available in health food stores and online, and all but no. 7, the IP-6, can be used for any immune disease you are fighting. Only use the IP-6 when fighting breast cancer, and consult a naturopathic doctor for additional supplements to combat other diseases.

Supplements

1. Vitamin C, you can use crystallized and add to juice and teas or tablets. Start with 1000mg a day and work your way up to 8,000mg. Vitamin C is water soluble, so any excess will be flushed out daily if it isn't used. Vitamin C prevents and fights free radicals, supporting the immune system.
2. Vitamin E – 1600mg – 1800mg a day is good in the fight. Vitamin C and E work well together; E is fat soluble and when both are taken simultaneously, they strengthen the benefits of the other.
3. Fish Oil (Omega 3s) at least 3000mg a day. Omega 3s will keep your arteries clear and flexible, so malformed cells cannot attach as easily to healthy cells. They also help clear out cholesterol and improve the heart function.
4. Selenium – 200mg x 2 times a day; super support for the immune system.

5. AHCC – is a mixture of mushrooms, which support the fighter cells in your system and enable them to attack the cancer cells. It demolishes and destroys them, so they can be flushed out. Take as directed.

6. Healthy Cell – take as directed. A mix of L-Lysine, L-Proline, L- Arginine, N-Acetyl Cysteine and Green Tea extract. This will strengthen the cellular structure of the cell walls, so it is more difficult for diseased cells to enter. (Peggy's Whole Foods, Daytona Beach, FL)

7. IP-6 – This supplement builds up cells and cell structure and comes in powder or capsule. It is especially for breast, prostate, and colon cells. The powder is difficult to mix, so try the capsules and follow the directions; take one capsule, 3x a day.

8. Co-Q 10 – 200mg – 300mg. Co-Q 10 is an excellent nutrient for blood circulation and the blood vessels. You need healthy blood cells because the bloodstream carries the crushed malformed cells out of the body.

9. Cat's Claw – 200mg. 2 or 3 times a day. This herb has been studied and found to fight cancer.

10. Barley or Alfalfa tablets – If your Ph level continues in the acidic range, try either of these to add more alkaline to the system. Barley and Alfalfa are both extremely alkaline-producing and should help balance your Ph level. Take 5 tablets, 3-4

times a day depending on how acidic your test is. (You cannot overdose on this.)

11. Black Cohosh – up to 600 mg a day. Has been researched and found to fight cancer. Start at 200 mg a day.

12. B Complex – 200 mg a day. Vitamin B helps digests proteins and brings a sense of calm by feeding the brain.

13. Vitamin D3 – If you can't get out in the sun for 20 minutes every day, take 400-600mg a day. Recent studies reveal that Vitamin D3 is the basis for cell restructuring and is the root of healing. 1,000 mg capsules is a healing dose.

14. Bromelain – 500 mg a day. This enzyme digests proteins very efficiently. Take 1 capsule on an empty stomach and the Bromelain will "eat up" leftover proteins in your system and clean your bloodstream. If you wake up in the middle of the night, take one with water, and go back to sleep. Let it work all night.

To raise your ph, Apple Cider Vinegar is extremely alkaline-producing, so add 2-3 tablespoons to salads for extra alkaline. ACV is good for a million things ranging from acid-reflux and stomach aches to joint and back pains, even easing arthritis. Google apple cider vinegar, and you'll see all the nutrients that are in this amazing natural product and why it is so good for you.

This is the list of supplements that I used to beat breast cancer. You may want to start out with one or two and work your way into all of them, but each of these have a specific purpose to kick cancer's butt. Within a month you should be taking all of them until you are cancer-free.

>>>

God is an Awesome God! You have read how He healed me, and how much better you're feeling by taking authority over disease and working to feed your body God's Way with God's natural foods. Keep believing and working the program because He loves you! If you would like to receive this healing God into your heart and life, it's all about a relationship with Him. You can know Him personally today. It is very simple. All it takes is an open heart and one sincere prayer.

Say this short prayer out loud from your heart:

"Father God,
Thank you for sending Your Son Jesus down to this earth to live and to die, but then to rise again for me. You are the perfect example of how I am to live on earth. Take away my sins and sicknesses as far as the east is from the west, so I can know You better. They stand in the way. Come into my heart and help me live my life.

I know You're real! You went to the cross and forgave me for everything I ever did against you; wash me clean!

Jesus, thank You for coming into my life. I know You love me, and because I know You, I will go to heaven. I am saved by the precious blood of Jesus from an eternity in hell. I am born again into Your Kingdom. I am a born-again child of God!

Thank you, Jesus! I know you have a plan for my life that is good. Thank You, God for Your Love, Life and Healing through Jesus. I'll love and follow You forever."

Read this out loud a few times. It's REAL! Jesus is alive and real!

Now you know John 3:16: For God so loved the world that He sent His only Son Jesus down to this earth that whosoever would believe in Him would not perish, but have everlasting life!

This would be a wonderful time to spend meditating on Jesus and His Goodness!

Part Two

Healing Your Soul and Spirit is a Lifestyle

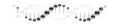

N ow you know what you can feed your body, it's time to send healing to your soul and spirit. The rest of the book will continue to do that, so it is essential for you to wrap your mind around Part Two.

Chapter 8

The Lost Art of Good Listening

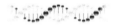

Your mind has quieted and you are adjusting to the right foods to eat ask yourself this question and give yourself an honest answer, "When was the last time I really listened to someone?" I know this sounds absurd, but what I mean is when did you totally surrender your agenda and actively listen to what someone was expressing? It could've been your husband or wife, another family member, a friend, someone at work, but whoever it was, you totally let them talk and you just listened without jumping in, correcting them or adding anything?

Now, do you remember what the result was? What happened when the two of you finished your conversation? Did you feel closer to that person? Do you think they felt any better? Maybe you both grew closer? But in any event, didn't it feel great to let someone share and connect with you?

Of course it did! When there is open communication shared between two human beings, it creates a spiritual bond. Even though your part might have been virtually non-verbal, you opened yourself up to their words, the inflection of their voice, and their body language, so you could understand what they were truly saying. If it's been awhile since you've given your full attention to someone's thoughts other than your own, you're due.

This is really something we all need to check ourselves on every so often. We are surrounded by people all day, and yet most of us can honestly say that we don't take the time to listen to each other. We hear, but we don't listen, but isn't it ironic that when we really need an answer, we pay close attention.

Think about it. We've all been in a strange city or a different part of town and gotten away from the directions for your destination, and now you're lost. What do you do? If you're a woman reading this, I know just what you'll do. You'll pull over to the nearest convenient store and ask how to get back on track again. And you'll listen intently, committing to memory what the person is saying because you really want to get back to familiar territory. If you're a man reading this – I have no idea what you'll do, since you don't ask for directions!

What I'm getting at is that in this hustle, bustle society Not many people take the time to listen (spiritually or physically) to someone else unless you need the information. Then we'll listen, but how many opportunities are missed in the interim?

Wouldn't it be great, if instead of running from this intimacy, we took some time every day to share with someone, maybe at the kitchen table with a glass of tea or in the breakroom at work, and give them 15 or 20 minutes as a gift to share what's going on in their life? We need to practice getting our own agendas out of the way and giving another person the chance to share how their day is going, what frustrated them today, what excited them, what are your thoughts about the country or the schools or the neighborhoods or whatever. The point is that by listening to them you are forgetting your own problems, while giving that person time to share what's important to them.

This allows them to share and be free of whatever might be bothering them, and then you have made two lives better by appreciating someone at a deeper level. Don't you agree that we could recover the lost art of conversation that is taking over the world today? That 15-20 minutes will improve relationships because there won't be the need to worry about the extra baggage that typically comes with free sharing; and you will be forgetting yourself. It's living life in the moment in its finest, so both parties feel immeasurably better.

This act of kindness is very meaningful to the person you're engaging with and it doesn't cost a thing. Maybe nobody ever takes the time to listen to them, and your active listening validated them for that day. We all need to feel heard and valued, and the 15-20 minutes you sacrificed at lunchtime has raised their acceptance level. It could bring a marriage back together or eliminate many of the endless disappointments that come from our emotions staying bottled up inside. And, if you're wondering what this has to do with your recovery from cancer, maybe sharing more every day would prevent those bottled up emotions from developing into cancer.

"Aha" - an Aha moment for so many. We all know that unexpressed emotions don't feel good, but feelings are not facts! They can change in a heart beat! Scientists have proven that keeping negative emotions and resentments that are bottled up causes the body to actually express them in the form of joint aches, high blood pressure, stomach and digestive problems and even cancer, just to name a few.

We have become a society that is closed and impersonal. Unforgiveness has also been researched and found to be the root cause of most diseases. Prolonged resentments and bitterness are not good for the mind, soul or body, so by opening up your being and listening and talking about whatever's bothering you every day, you eliminate those negative emotions and lift the weight of them off your shoulders. Your body is going to thank you.

The 20th-century farmer talked to everyone he met all day long, and the culture had very little cancer. The

21st-century businessman or woman is moving so fast through the day that they don't open up to anyone. If we would talk to our family and neighbors, the bitterness that gets trapped inside and creates darkness and disease would begin to dissipate and the malformed cells would not form as rapidly or maybe not at all.

Science has proven that the resentment a person holds builds walls in their souls, which buries those emotions and thoughts deep inside where they continue to grow and fester. So, if cancer is found in the body, darkness that is trapped needs to find a way out. Forgiveness is the only way to release those pent-up emotions. The soul has its home in the body, so whatever is felt in the soul is manifested in the body. Let Go and Let God! Everyone on the planet has similar housing, so unforgiveness and resentment have to be released to have peace and healing.

Eliminating "Stuffed Emotions"

Research shows that stuffing your emotions and feelings and not sharing them is the major cause of our anxieties today. Listening to people share what's on their minds is a fantastic way to relieve some of the stress.

Here are four ways to release pent-up emotions and bring Light into your soul, so your body can heal. Try one or all of these suggestions whether you think this applies to you or not. It is better to know that you have brought forgiveness into your life than to go on walking around like a time bomb waiting to explode. And before the explosion occurs, and it will, it will contribute to feeding the cancer in the body.

1. Keep a journal, and write in it regularly especially when situations are bothering you. Writing releases tension and anxiety. Writing a letter to express emotions that you've been holding back, whether good or bad, will help release pent-up feelings. If you are really at odds with the person, write the letter and say everything you honestly want to say, and then tear it up! You will still reap the benefits of releasing the stress, but they will never have to hear it. It is surprising how much better you'll feel by releasing emotions properly and with forgiveness.

2. Take a walk every day, and allow God to bring to the surface anything that is deep down inside. Talk it out with Him outloud! Let people think you're crazy – it keeps them wondering! The walk will also improve your circulation and keep your energy level up.

3. If you like massages, they are an incredible way to release tension and stress that gets locked inside your muscles and joints. Afterward, soak in a hot tub with Frankincense oil, and you'll feel 100% human again.

4. Get a dog or a cat, and pet it often. Studies show that people who have pets have less stress than people who don't and consequently live longer. Petting releases physical stress.

Getting More Involved

Now back to listening. When you are intently listening, it is called "active listening;" and you are using all of your senses, not just your ears. You are listening with your ears, but your eyes are watching the body language and your mind is memorizing every word. Think back to the example of being lost where you are actively listening and absorbing everything the store clerk is saying as they are giving directions. You are listening to their words, but you are watching their body language intently, (they could be pointing out to the street or in a certain direction). Then you might even repeat what they said back to them to make sure you got it right. Psychology recognizes this as active listening, and by doing this, your communication is bound to improve because you are focusing and using more of your senses.

When I need an answer, I use all the resources that I have access to. When I heard the words that my surgeon said as he expressed my diagnosis of multi-focal breast cancer, my heart stopped. That is the power of speaking words. He talked and I listened, but I was also watching his eyes and his body language because the information was so important to me.

Reaching Out

I began to tune in to others who had been through cancer, and I started to search for information that would apply to me. I'm sure many of you who are in this fight have called the National Cancer Society to see how they can assist you. This is a start.

You might have been referred to cancer survivors who were willing to talk about their experiences. I know my doctor gave me a list of several survivors in my area, so I contacted a few of these women, but they left me wanting more. I wasn't ready to settle for their experiences and what they had settled with. I went online and began to research many different avenues people had taken to be healed and to prevent the drastic treatments the doctor had planned. I was determined to turn this thing around, and God was on my side, just like He is with you.

I researched nutrients and vitamins and found out which ones were beneficial in attacking the cancer in different areas of the body. Both my church and my community had cancer support groups where survivors shared their stories and offered their support. These allowed me to open up about the things that were on my mind. I couldn't let it stay bottled up inside, and they allowed me to share while they shared the hope they had.

One thing I noticed though, was that everyone I met who went through the fight with cancer emerges with a special strength and desire to help others. It is really beautiful to see how one person reaches out to another who is still suffering and shares their victory. No matter how serious you think your case is, you will see that your experience will benefit others. Hang in there! More will be revealed.

There is an incredible amount of information on cancer, so you have to be extremely discerning in what you accept as truth. Keep an open mind and stick close to the book. There is a lot of flaky information online that must be evaluated and verified before it can be used, but you can rest assured that everything in this book is rooted in science.

Because of this disease, I now have a friend who is the owner of a health food store in my town, and he is a doctor of naturopathy. This practice does not use chemicals for healing, they use natural products that allows the body to heal itself. I found I could trust him to verify questions that I had about products I was unsure of. It is extremely important to have new information verified, but new techniques in natural healing come out every month. Look for someone in the holistic or natural health fields, such as a nutritionist or a doctor of naturopathy.

Changing my mindset has caused me to overcome this deadly disease. If I had remained satisfied to accept the disease as a physical malady with only a physical solution, I probably would not have defeated the enemy permanently. Pay attention to everything you hear and read, but filter it to see if you can use it in your healing. The last chapter would be a good place to start. There are a number of websites where you can begin your own research. I listed websites that are packed with information, and then provided recipes for snacks and meals for your everyday meals. You'll love it, and you won't need to go anywhere else unless you want to.

With that said, this is not the time to isolate yourself in the house because the negative thoughts will only multiply and affect your emotions. Keep your ears and eyes open to everything. I knew there had to be a natural way to recover because the human body is designed to heal itself. I knew there was an alternative answer to chemo and radiation. The Creator surely has a plan to heal the bodies He created. The Word says that "all things work together for good to those who love Him......All Things, even the not-so-good things. Romans 8:28

Many years ago, I heard the saying that I should learn something new every day. It still sounds like an excellent ideal to me, so whatever I am experiencing today, I see what can be learned in it. It only makes sense.

I watched videos on breast cancer and nutrition, ways to prevent cancer, the necessity of the right antioxidants and strengthening the immune system because a damaged immune system is the root of most diseases. I studied women's health both online and in magazines. All these things began to work together, and I'm so grateful that I stopped and took the time to see a world beyond the doctor's office because that's what it took. Life with blinders is not for me. Change is uncomfortable at times, but it's going to happen. Get your support from a variety of sources. The Word says to "get counsel from many sources," so you have a better source of information. There are many success stories out there.

Father God wants to you to come in from the world of chaos that is going on in the world today, and just sit down and rest. You can tell Him what your day's been like, and believe it or not, He listens to everyone on the planet. He'll listen for as long as you need Him too, and then when you are finished talking, He takes advantage of your stillness and begins to talk to you.

Be still and know that I am God. Ruwach. When you calm your inner self from somewhere, deep inside your consciousness, comes the still quiet voice of the Father, steady and sure. Whether you thought you believed in a Higher Presence or not, He is there. Now, you can really begin to use your listening skills. It might not happen the first or second time you get still, but the more you become comfortable with being quiet and taking the time to listen, the more you'll find He's been right there all along. He will give you an impression for the next right thing to do.

Taking Action

Listening to your innermost self is vital at this point. If you're having trouble slowing your mind and body down, try one of these easy exercises. They will stop the tapes from going around in your mind that say things like "you know people die from cancer" or "why are you doing this natural stuff, it's not strong enough!" When you do any type of exercise, focus on the activity and listen to your breathing or sing and shout to music, whatever makes you feel good and gets your mind off yourself.

Exercise works so well because it accelerates your heart rate and forces more cancer cells out of your body as long as you are eating well and drinking lots of filtered water and tea. Then after a hot shower, the voice of your problems may quiet down to a manageable state.

If you can take a walk, do that. Walking is known as the perfect body exercise along with swimming. Nothing in these exercises is difficult, and if the weather's nice, it will allow you to get outside and focus on the blue sky or something else positive, but you can't keep the depressing thoughts in your mind.

Don't do anything that causes pain, but find a way to raise your heart rate and keep your system stimulated for 15 minutes every day. As you find more ways to support your system and promote good health, you will demolish more of the diseased cells that are residing in your body uninvited. It's all about fighting back: feeding

the recovery and starving the disease. This is the cycle
to continue until you have won.

One of the most effective methods for stimulating
your system is stationary breathing exercises. These are
perfect to do while you are lying on a couch or a bed.
Take about 15 minutes at the beginning and end of your
day or do them as often as you like. You cannot overdose
on them! They will allow you to unwind and your body
to fall into its instinctual rhythm, which will allow more
oxygen in your blood. These exercises will motivate your
circulation, and release tension.

Real Breathing Exercises

Breathing exercises are a must if you are fighting the
fight, so add them to your schedule. You just may find
that you like doing them so much that you do them even
after the cancer is gone; they are so easy and relaxing.
Winners in every sport know they have to put aside time
for themselves, so here you go. This time is for you.

Lie down on a flat comfortable surface and stretch
out; reach as high as you can above your head with both
arms while stretching out your legs all the way to your
toes. Then, relax and bring your arms down to your sides.

Now, begin by taking a breath that fills your lower
abdomen and stomach, and then fill your lungs and chest.
Hold that fresh, new air in for about six seconds, and
then slowly release, pushing all the air out. Inhale slowly

again and repeat; do this slowly for at least 15 minutes. You'll begin to feel your entire system come into sync as you take in full lungs of fresh oxygen that goes straight into your bloodstream.

The new oxygen that you are taking in is instantly absorbed through the lungs and transmitted into the blood. It is then circulated by the bloodstream feeding all of your live cells with the fresh oxygen. This is extremely important because cancer cells cannot live in an oxygenated environment, so by bringing in the fresh air, the malformed cells are being suffocated while the healthy cells are absorbing the fresh oxygen and gaining strength. Did you ever think breathing could do so much for you? Fresh air is vital for a healthy life.

As you are breathing, concentrate on the oxygen as it is filling every organ in your body. Imagine it going deep, deep down inside and then reaching out into every part of the body that God made for you. Try to focus on how your body is responding as you inhale, and then slowly release it. The old saying goes "a picture is worth a thousand words," so picture your live cells - healthy, round, red and perfect. Your tissue is pink and healthy, full of oxygen.

Many studies on the brain show that it registers positive images by creating positive physical reactions, so by switching your focus to the LIFE in your body and the benefits of fresh air, and not the disease, your stress and worry will decrease. Remind yourself that it's going to be OK. You are in the Hands of the Creator, and He died so that you could live.

Do your breathing exercises twice a day, and in only a few days, you'll notice 1) how much better you're feeling and 2) how you look forward to your quiet meditation time. I know I did!

There is one more benefit if you can stand it, and it could be the most important. If you are taking deep breaths and concentrating on the life you are generating, then you are naturally quieting your mind, soul, and body. This is another perfect place to listen. Listen to your breathing. Listen to the way your body reacts to fresh, deliberate breaths, and listen to soft music if you like, and, if you turn everything off and listen to the stillness, you just might hear the sounds of silence encouraging you on.

To make this breathing time more meaningful, take a few minutes after you're done to rest and allow yourself to slip into prayer. Prayer is nothing more than a conversation with God. Talk to Him about your healing, pray for guidance, pray for your family or others around you, you just want to keep a connection with the Healer. You may feel silly at first "talking to yourself," but this is the best way to get your answers, and you may have been doing it for years.

If you need some more subjects to pray for: pray for peace in the U.S., pray for lives saved and ask God to bless America and the world again. Talk about your feelings or this fight you are participating in. It is OK to pray for yourself? Of course, it is. Ask God if there's anybody he wants you to help today? Forgive everyone you can think of because life's too short to hold on to all that negativity, and ask Him if there's anything He wants you to do to beat the enemy of cancer. Now listen for the answers.

It was during these times, where I first got the impression to write this book, Cancer, then no cancer! God had more faith in me than I had for myself, and yet, here it is, and you've read more than half! It's real! This praying atmosphere is also a healing one, so stay in it as long as possible remembering that now you know how to reach this quiet zone, and you can come back anytime.

What's in Your Kitchen?

When I first got home from the doctor after hearing the diagnosis, I just collapsed on the sofa. I rested for a long time. God quieted my mind, and I wanted to get busy recovering! I went into the kitchen and began emptying out the cabinets of all the poison foods that were in there. I knew they were the problem. All the foods I loved had gotten me into this mess, and my cabinets and refrigerator were filled with them. They had poisoned my body to the point of this diagnosis.

I tossed out everything that had these ingredients: sugar, flour, anything with chemicals, steroids, and preservatives. If it was one of the ingredients listed on the label, I put it in the big, black garbage bags to get out of my house. These ingredients were in the foods I ate every day, and I had been feeding the cancerous cells without knowing it. My plan in recovery was to starve the malformed cells out by taking away their fuel, the toxic foods.

This is the ultimate goal I started with - to starve the cancer cells out. Everything else in this book is connected to that concept. I gave away two big garbage bags of food that I couldn't eat anymore. I'm not sure who really can, but they're not for me any longer.

Next, I began a quest to investigate why these foods were poison for someone with cancer, and it was amazingly simple - they are poison to everyone, but some of us are more susceptible than others. Sugar is the first, and foremost food to eliminate if you need healing. If you do nothing else for your recovery, stop eating white sugar, aka delicious donuts, cakes, cookies, ice cream, candy, white bread. Anything made with sugar is food for the cancer cells to consume and then multiply. Flour is not allowed while you are fighting, either, because flour converts to sugar during digestion and also causes bacteria growth, which gives malformed cells a comfy environment to reproduce in.

These are our favorite foods, but they are also cancer cell's favorites! The more you eat these, the more cancer cells multiply; eliminate them, and you are fighting and reducing the disease. This handbook teaches a successful way to starve the malformed cells to death and wash them out quickly. This is the goal. If you are reading this book for any other reason, other diseased cells will be destroyed and new cells will be strengthened. Feeding the malformed cells in your body with sugar leads to other diseases, so don't push this information aside. Consider and act.

Chemicals and preservatives in food speak loudly for themselves. They are toxic to everyone with a disease and to those who are totally healthy! All diseases feed on these poisons, and like my mother said to me more than once growing up, "Just because everybody else is doing it, doesn't make it right."

So, why does the American public continue to keep eating food that is creating chronic diseases? Because they are not aware of the consequences, and because they are so convenient. They are EVERYWHERE. You must make a conscious decision to avoid them, at all costs. And, it takes awhile, so give yourself a learning curve.

This is a good place to note that the sweet flavor in fruit is a natural sugar called fructose and because since it is naturally produced in the fruit itself, it is not detrimental to your health like white sugar and artificial sugars. For those fighting cancer, though, three or four servings a day is enough. Keep it in moderation because the body is still going to store any excess sugar that isn't used right away. The malformed cells have easy access to anything that is stored.

Chapters 5, 6 and 7 go into more detail about the foods to eat and those you should avoid.

Check back and see what is in those chapters. This is a handbook, so you can use it like that. Not to worry, this natural way of eating will get easier as you go on.

Chapter 9

As You Keep Listening, Your Spirit Gets Stronger

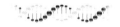

You're walking in the Sonlight of the Spirit now, and you are going to find new hope every day. From the deep breathing exercises and finding a quiet state of rest to clearing the junk food out of the cupboards. Every positive action you take is allowing the Light to shine brighter in you. You were created to be healthy and full of life and that is exactly where you're headed. Keep that in your mind always, and never let others tell you differently. You're a WINNER, and you will succeed, too! You might have to take a vacation from some of the negative people in your life who are distracting you from a positive recovery, but you can invite them back when you are totally cancer free and recovered.

Listening to negative words and attitudes damages the positive atmosphere you are building, no matter who is saying them. If they are not speaking Life, Love and Victory to you, you might have to avoid them until you are well, even if those people are part of your family. God wants you surrounded with positive words that create a positive, spiritual atmosphere.

Kindly tell them you are working on something, on your healing. Don't listen to their comments about being sick and getting worse and dying because these options are not for you. I also suggest telling as few people as possible about your diagnosis, and then you won't have to provide as many answers. Your job is to stay positive. You're a winner, I'm a winner and together we make a Winning Team!

I stayed with those who had encouraging words to say. From the very beginning, God told me to take a year to focus on my recovery, and I would be completely healed. He is no respecter of persons - He will do the same for you, as He did for me. God can heal you any way He wants to!

The time it takes to be completely healed and cancer-free will differ for each individual, so don't count the days. For me, it took less than six months because it was at my regularly scheduled six-month mammogram that I was declared cancer-free. The cancer was benign. What is more important than counting days is to change your lifestyle to a healthy and caregiving one that will lead to being cancer-free. I have not gone back to my old way of living since I learned this immune-building, cancer-preventing, natural way of life. I have more energy and more focus than I ever imagined possible. It is amazing!

My life has improved incredibly; I feel 100% healthier than I ever was. This lifestyle is the nutritional way to bring your body into vibrant health. It is an extremely fulfilling way to live, so there is no reason for me to give it up. I don't miss any of the "death foods" I was so used to eating, and if I keep up the plan I've shared with you, then there is a 94% chance that no cancer of any kind will return to my body.

The other benefits, besides becoming cancer-free, include lowering high blood pressure and high cholesterol, eliminating RA arthritis, losing 16 pounds and improving my skin tone and condition. Yes, this way of life allows me to be more creative with my everyday diet and to enjoy its life-giving benefits.

40 Scriptures 4 You

Having a conversation with God is best to do in your own words. There are no pretenses with the Father, but allow me to offer this list of super-strong healing Scriptures because they are the words of God that stop the disease in its tracks and secure healing. They are a wonderful tool to use daily to create that healthy, positive atmosphere in your home. They are a contradiction to the negativity that surrounds any disease. Reading the list out loud presents a spiritual attack on the disease, and remember, for your recovery to be successful, it must include healing of your spirit, soul and body. These Scriptures are spiritual words, straight out of the Bible. If you don't really get them the first time you read through, you will. Give them time.

Since, every disease needs to be fought and won on a mental, emotional, physical, and spiritual level, bombarding this evil disease with good, positive and healing words from The Word is the solution to any issue or sickness you have. I have listed them in their entirety, and you can print them out for easier access.

I read this list outloud every day, twice a day, and the reason I incorporated them into my recovery is so I would be sure to have something positive flowing into my life. The Dead Sea has no life in it because it does not allow water to flow in and out. God's life-giving words coming into our lives is the best. As a side benefit, they bring peace to you as you read them, so reading them at night before you go to sleep and in the morning after breakfast are the times that worked for me.

They are a spiritually strong way to begin and end the day. Turn off the crime shows, mystery movies, and the news, which are filled with violence and murder, and instill fear into your mind. The last images you see or read before you fall asleep are the ones that replay in your subconscious as you sleep. Wouldn't you rather be putting positive words into your spirit and soul to create a foundation of hope and love to build your faith?

NKJV stands for New King James Version, but there are many translations of the Bible, and you can find the one that fits your personality by looking on BibleGateway.com.

1. The Word of God will save your life. "My son, give attention to my words; Incline your ear to my sayings. Do not let them depart from your eyes; Keep them in the midst of your heart. For they are life to those who find them and health to all their flesh." (Proverbs 4:20-22)
2. God's Word will not fail. "Not a word failed of any good thing which the LORD had spoken to the house of Israel. All came to pass." (Joshua 21:45)
3. God's will of healing is working in you. "For it is God who works in you both to will and to do for His good pleasure." (Philippians 2:13)
4. The Spirit of Life is making your body alive. "But if the Spirit of Him who raised Jesus from the dead dwells in you, He who raised Christ from the dead will also give life to your mortal bodies through His Spirit who dwells in you." (Romans 8:11)
5. God is for you. "For all the promises of God in Him are Yes, and in Him Amen to the glory of God through us." (2 Corinthians 1:20)

6. It is God's will for you to be healed. "And behold, a leper came and worshipped Him, saying, 'Lord, if You are willing, You can make me clean.' Then Jesus put out His hand and touched him, saying, 'I am willing; be cleansed.' Immediately his leprosy was cleansed." (Matthew 8:2-3)

7. Obey God's Word and be healed. "If you diligently heed the voice of the LORD your God and do what is right in His sight, give ear to His commandments and keep all His statutes, I will put none of the diseases on you which I have brought on the Egyptians. For I am the LORD who heals you." (Exodus 15:26)

8. Serve the Lord and healing will be yours. "So you shall serve the LORD your God, and He will bless your bread and your water. And I will take sickness away from the midst of you." (Exodus 23:25)

9. God takes all sickness away from you. "And the LORD will take away from you all sickness, and will afflict you with none of the terrible diseases of Egypt which you have known, but will lay them on all those who hate you." (Deuteronomy 7:15)

10. Obey all God's commandments and receive all His blessings. "'Bring all the tithes into the storehouse, that there may be food in My house, and try Me now in this,' Says the LORD of hosts, 'If I will not open for you the windows of heaven and

pour out for you such blessing that there will not be room enough to receive it.'" (Malachi 3:10)

11. One of God's benefits is healing. "Bless the LORD, O my soul; And all that is within me, bless His holy name. Bless the LORD, O my soul, and forget not all His benefits: Who forgives all your iniquities, Who heals all your diseases, Who redeems your life from destruction, Who crowns you with loving-kindness and tender mercies, Who satisfies your mouth with good things, So that your youth is renewed like the eagle's." (Psalms 103:1-5)

12. God's Word is healing. "He sent His word and healed them, and delivered them from their destructions." (Psalms 107:20)

13. God wants you to live. "I shall not die, but live, and declare the works of the LORD." (Psalms 118:17)

14. Choose to live. Be a fighter! "I call heaven and earth as witnesses today against you that I have set before you life and death, blessing and cursing; therefore choose life, that both you and your descendants may live." (Deuteronomy 30:19)

15. You will live a long life. "With long life I will satisfy him, and show him My salvation." (Psalms 91:16)

16. Jesus bore your sins AND your sicknesses. "But He was wounded for our transgressions, He was bruised for our iniquities; The chastisement for

our peace was upon Him, And by His stripes, we are healed." (Isaiah 53:5)

17. God will restore your health. "'For I will restore health to you and heal you of your wounds,' says the LORD, 'Because they called you an outcast saying: 'This is Zion; No one seeks her.'" (Jeremiah 30:17)

18. You can take authority over the sickness in your body. "Assuredly, I say to you, whatever you bind on earth will be bound in heaven, and whatever you loose on earth will be loosed in heaven." (Matthew 18:18)

19. Agree with someone for your healing. "Again I say to you that if two of you agree on earth concerning anything that they ask, it will be done for them by My Father in heaven." (Matthew 18:19)

20. What you say will make a difference. "So Jesus answered and said to them, 'Have faith in God. For assuredly, I say to you, whoever says to this mountain, 'Be removed and be cast into the sea,' and does not doubt in his heart, but believes that those things he says will be done, he will have whatever he says." (Mark 11:22-23)

21. Believe, and you will receive. "Therefore, I say to you, whatever things you ask when you pray, believe that you receive them, and you will have them."(Mark 11:24)

22. Plead your case before God. "Even I am He who blots out your transgressions for My own sake, And I will not remember your sins. Put Me in remembrance; Let us contend together; State your case, that you may be acquitted." (Isaiah 43:25-26)

23. Have someone lay hands on you for healing. "And these signs will follow those who believe: In My name they will cast out demons; they will speak with new tongues; they will take up serpents; and if they drink anything deadly, it will by no means hurt them; they will lay hands on the sick, and they will recover." (Mark 16:17-18)

24. Worship God. "If anyone is a worshiper of God and does His will, He hears him." (John 9:31)

25. The devil wants to kill you; God wants to heal you. "The thief does not come except to steal, and to kill, and to destroy. I have come that they may have life, and that they may have it more abundantly." (John 10:10)

26. You are redeemed from the curse. "Christ has redeemed us from the curse of the law, having become a curse for us (for it is written, 'Cursed is everyone who hangs on a tree') that the blessing of Abraham might come upon the Gentiles in Christ Jesus, that we might receive the promise of the Spirit through faith." (Galatians 3:13-14)

27. You will not waiver in your faith. "Let us hold fast the confession of our hope without wavering, for He who promised is faithful." (Hebrews 10:23)

28 You can have confidence in God and His Word. "Therefore, do not cast away your confidence, which has great reward." (Hebrews 10:35)

29. You can find strength in God and His Word. "Let the weak say, 'I am strong.'" (Joel 3:10)

30. Jesus Christ has never changed, and He never will. What He did in the Bible, He will do for you today. "Jesus Christ is the same yesterday, today, and forever." (Hebrews 13:8)

31. God's highest wish is for you to be well. "Beloved, I wish above all things that you would prosper and be in health even as thy soul prospers." (3 John 1:2 KJV)

32. Be anointed with oil by a Christian who believes in healing. "Is anyone among you sick? Let him call for the elders of the church, and let them pray over him, anointing him with oil in the name of the Lord. And the prayer of faith will save the sick, and the Lord will raise him up. And if he has committed sins, he will be forgiven." (James 5:14-15)

33. Jesus has already paid the price for your healing. "Who Himself bore our sins in His own body on the tree, that we, having died to sins, might live for righteousness; by whose stripes you were healed." (1 Peter 2:24)

34. Be confident in your prayers. "Now this is the confidence that we have in Him, that if we ask anything according to His will, He hears us. And if we know that He hears us, whatever we ask, we know that we have the petitions that we have asked of Him." (1 John 5:14-15)

35. God answers the prayers of those that keep His commandments. "Beloved, if our heart does not condemn us, we have confidence toward God. And whatever we ask we receive from Him, because we keep His commandments and do those things that are pleasing in His sight." (1 John 3:21-22)

36. Fear is not of God. Rebuke it! "For God has not given us a spirit of fear, but of power and of love and of a sound mind." (2 Timothy 1:7)

37. Cast down those thoughts and imaginations that don't line up with the Word of God. "For the weapons of our warfare are not carnal but mighty in God for pulling down strongholds, casting down arguments and every high thing that exalts itself against the knowledge of God, bringing every thought into captivity to the obedience of Christ." (2 Corinthians 10:4-5)

38. Be strong in the Lord's power. Put on His armor to fight for healing. "Finally, my brethren, be strong in the Lord and in the power of His might. Put on the whole armor of God that you may be able to stand against the wiles of the devil. For we

do not wrestle against flesh and blood, but against principalities, against powers, against the rulers of the darkness of this age, against spiritual hosts of wickedness in the heavenly places. Therefore, take up the whole armor of God that you may be able to withstand in the evil day, and having done all, to stand. Stand therefore, having girded your waist with truth, having put on the breastplate of righteousness, and having shod your feet with the preparation of the gospel of peace; above all, taking the shield of faith with which you will be able to quench all the fiery darts of the wicked one. And take the helmet of salvation and the sword of the Spirit, which is the word of God." (Ephesian 6:10)

39. Give testimony of your healing. "And they overcame him by the blood of the Lamb and by the word of their testimony, and they did not love their lives to the death." (Revelation 12:11)

40. Your sickness will leave and not come back again. "What do you conspire against the LORD? He will make an utter end of it. Affliction will not rise up a second time." (Nahum 1:9)

Sleep well. If you are fighting cancer, you need 8-10 hours of deep REM sleep so your body can detoxify every night. Scientists tell us that the hours you sleep before midnight give you double the value. Therefore, if you go to sleep at 10 pm, you get two hours worth double or the equivalent of four hours of recovery sleep until midnight. The old saying stands true: "Early to bed, early to rise, makes a man/woman healthy, wealthy, and wise." I tried to be in bed by 10 PM every night and slept until 8 AM.

Remember, prayer is simply connecting in conversation with the Father. When you want to talk to Him, use the language He understands - your everyday language, and wait for answers. You simply need to be still and let the connection begin. Blessing your food at meals is another time you can let God into your day by just saying "Thank You!"

Here's a short prayer:

"Father God, bless this food and let it be used for Your will in my life. Thank you."

Just say it to yourself, that's enough. For some people, this will be a traumatic change in habits to stop during the daily routine and recognize the Creator as God in your day. It will allow you to get out of yourself and direct your attention away from the disease. Taking 25 seconds of prayer before you eat is enough to remind you the Higher Power is ready and able to lead the way.

Breaking old eating habits is a major part of fighting the disease. When you allow God in, you're letting the disease know that it is not in control, and it cannot win.

Prayer is addressing the spiritual. Your new trend of clean, healthy natural eating will affect you mentally, emotionally and physically, and the mealtime blessing will bring in the spiritual by giving credit to God. This may be something you've never thought about before, but you feed all four areas when you have a meal.

God's Word is probably the most important element of this whole manual. If you don't already have a Bible, you can get one in any bookstore for $7.99 to $199 or at a Thrift store for less. Check out different translations because, in 2017, Bibles are written in every style of speech such as New International, New American, The Message or the New Living Word.

The reason the Bible is so important is that it is your guidebook for life. The stories are true, they simply occurred in a different time, but they adapt to any time and any culture. You have an instruction book from the manufacturer of your car, don't you? Well, God gave us a manual because He is our Creator. He knows everything about us and loves us anyway.

The Bible applies to all the circumstances in your life. As you read the words, starting in the New Testament with Matthew, Mark, Luke, and John, you'll see how much He really knows and loves you. John writes all about His Love. Read a portion of it every day, and you will begin to understand more and more as you read. Guaranteed. Know the Truth, and the Truth will set you Free!

Chapter 10

Talk the Talk, Walk the Walk

Talking the Talk

Hopefully, you are enjoying your deep breathing exercises in the morning and evening. The glory of having this handbook is that you can go back to any section, anytime and review. The book tells the whole story and offers a proven clear path to follow, and I am completely healthy! Light shines at the end of the tunnel and more will be revealed the more you read. Cancer Free are two of the best words you'll ever hear.

For me, I had to learn as much as possible about the nature of cancer, so I spent long periods of time online and at my local health food/supplement store. I asked questions and a good store is always happy to answer any questions or direct you to another source if they needed to. You might not have the inquisitive, perfectionist mindset that I had, but that is why I put all the information into this one source.

I began to discover what I needed to fight cancer and recover, and then maintained my health. As coincidence would have it, I had enrolled in an online nutrition course in 2006, and I used that information immediately. This would prove to be one of the best sources I had. The course taught me all the basics including how to strengthen the immune system, drinking filtered water, the vitamins and minerals I needed to get back to optimum health and how to use natural foods to benefit the fight.

I began to develop a completely new way of thinking as I progressed. My mind was opened and my thinking became more flexible. The AMA treats disease with a Band-aid mentality, but this natural treatment program was attacking the root of the cancer at the cellular level. I learned that my body is perfectly able to recreate itself if it is given the proper nutrition. Family DNA and genealogy can even be overcome with the right diet and supplements.

This natural or holistic approach is as foreign to the medical profession as night is to day. The medical profession is taught only to treat symptoms, while holistic medicine treats the causes and roots as well as the symptoms. For this reason, "Cancer, then no cancer" is filled with nutritional habits and lifestyle changes that bring healing.

Treating the root causes not only cures the disease, but when the root is eliminated in the body, mind, soul, and spirit, it is eradicated for good and won't come back. Pills and prescriptions only mask the problem and reduce the symptoms. It is interesting to note that the natural solutions can work right alongside the medical to bring healing results faster and more complete.

In the case of cancer, with the dangerous use of chemo and radiation, which is proven to destroy both the good and the bad cells, these treatments can be improved with a natural power-packed lifestyle. Most doctors steer away from natural health because they don't know how the body uses nutrients to rejuvenate and restore, and this is a tragedy for the American public.

To get a holistic or drug-free perspective, see a doctor of naturopathy, an ND or a nutritionist. Naturopathic doctors are trained in accredited, 4-year, post-graduate, residential naturopathic medical programs. To date, only 16 states and the District of Columbia recognize them for medical practice, but that is slowly changing.

The Footwork

Now, it's time to quit talking the talk and start really walking the walk. I gave everything to this fight because it had everything; there was no holding back. The first thing I did was get several large plastic garbage bags and started getting rid of everything in the cupboards that was on my list of cancer instigators: sugar, flour, and all the foods with chemicals and preservatives. Preservatives are all those long names I couldn't pronounce. I read the ingredients on each package and every label, every bag of chips, boxes of macaroni and cheese and broccoli with cheese sauce, crackers, cookies, noodles, soup – Everything! And I tossed most of it into the bag. I refer to these as fake foods because there is nothing living in them. They are dead and will only produce death. I filled an entire garbage bag.

The refrigerator was next, and when I was finished, I had two huge garbage bags full of the cancer-causing foods I had been eating all my life. It was dead food that I could no longer eat safely, so I would give it to someone with a better immune system than mine. I'm betting that the majority of Americans can't handle those foods, either, so that's why our cancer and disease rates are skyrocketing. They're toxic foods, poison, and I don't want them in my body any longer.

When it was all said and done, what remained was a box of Minute Brown Rice, grits, oatmeal and a container of vanilla protein powder. In the refrigerator, I had a bottle of natural cranberry juice, a few bags of frozen broccoli, a container of soy milk, a half jar of salsa, two sticks of butter and a jar of pickles. My new life begins here.

I was getting rid of the old, and I felt empowered. I gave both bags to someone who could use them; I had made a decision to start with a clean slate. The unhealthy food wasn't for me anymore – it was trying to kill me! By cleaning out my kitchen, I was making a tremendous statement towards my new lifestyle. Old things were passing away, and all things were becoming new. I was moving into better health by leaps and bounds, and this was an incredible step forward on the path of victory.

I suggest that you do the same thing; it will make a statement both to yourself and to those around you. It was a Spectacular First Step!

First Shopping Trip for Nutritious Food

Then, I got dressed and went shopping. I was determined to stock up with all the good foods I could find. I was about to discover foods that would give my body a fighting chance, and surprisingly, I would enjoy. So, let's keep walking..........

The Alkaline Food List in chapter 6 is the list to take with you when you go food shopping, so you can get used to identifying the healthier foods. The list plainly divides the foods into two groups: alkaline and acid. Focus on the alkaline-producing foods to put in your cart because research has shown that disease cannot grow in an alkaline environment. The disease is literally snuffed out because the germs and bacteria cells of sickness need higher acidity levels to grow and thrive. Sickness and inflammation is the result of eating acid-producing foods such as packaged food, junk food, and fast food.

As you are shopping, you will also use a skill that up until now you may have been neglecting and that is looking for key facts on the labels of the foods before you purchase them, The FDA requires all packages to have certain information, such as fiber, sugar and sodium content. Learning to read labels is imperative when you are fighting cancer or working at other diseases, so you are aware of what you are actually consuming. The FDA also requires by law that every ingredient is listed from top to bottom in order of the percentage of each ingredient that was in the product. So, the first ingredient has the most, and the last ingredient has the least.

If you purchase all organic, label reading will not take as long because organic products by definition are made with products that have been grown, harvested and shipped using no chemicals, steroids or pesticides. You know from the start that the ingredients are clean and chemical-free, from packaged foods to meats and cheeses.

"Clean foods" are defined as those foods that contain none of the toxic ingredients mentioned and none were used in the processing or packaging. This is the way you are going to be eating. Local farmers do not use as many pesticides as national growers who ship fruits and vegetables, so you can easily shop your local produce market for fresh fruits and vegetables that are less expensive and know that they have fewer pesticides on them. Always wash all fresh foods thoroughly.

Organic is the safest way to buy, if possible, but it is not always necessary. If you read labels and buy locally, you'll generally find simpler foods.

FYI - "Natural products" are defined as natural foods that were not submitted to pesticides and other chemicals, and they are also whole foods like apples and grapes that were grown and shipped with no chemicals or other additives. Natural and organic foods are what you want to look for.

The only products you must purchase organic are the animal products – meats, cheeses, and eggs. These must be clean and organic while you are fighting the battle because animals raised for wholesale are injected with steroids and hormones in the U.S. to make them grow larger, faster. They are not fed natural foods or treated with dignity, so you don't want to support that method anyway. Purchase meat that has labels that use these words, "Natural, no added flavorings, no steroids, no preservatives, Grass-fed, or Organic. These are all good signs about the quality of the product. Fish should Not say "farm raised;" It should be "wild-caught."

Have as much protein as you like because it is so essential to your health in these forms, and don't forget whey protein shakes. Norwegian Seafood is optimum when purchasing fish because these are caught in clean, pristine waters, which have no pollution. These fish have abundant levels of Omega 3s besides being an excellent source of protein. On any given day, you want to aim for 40-90 grams of protein because protein is found in every cell of the body.

Cow's milk and cheeses are definitely off limits for the above reasons and because dairy products cause bacteria growth in the intestines. You don't want bacteria growth at all in your body, especially when fighting cancer. (see milk research and cancer in chapter 7) Stick to Almond or rice milk or goats milk, if your health food store carries the fresh variety. Always buy natural organic cheeses, if you must have them. Remove cow's milk from your life!

The goal is to feed the good cells and starve the malformed cells, right? And the good cells far out-number the bad.

Shopping

So, I left for the grocery store and began to shop like a madwoman, but a smart, healthy-minded madwoman. Most of the foods that you'll want are those around the perimeter of the store: the produce section, deli, meat department, refrigerated sections. Typically, the natural and organic sections are placed around the walls of stores with the freezers and refrigerators. All the processed and packaged foods are in the center aisles, so you won't need much from there, maybe rice, grits, and oatmeal.

When you enter the store, go straight to the health food section to see what you can find there first. Enough sitting around; let's get into some positive action and walk the talk of healing and success. Simply look for foods you think you like and those you'd like to try. With your alkaline and acidic list in hand, shop with health and taste in mind, walking around the perimeter.

The next stop is the local produce market and health food store in your area. If you are lucky enough to have a grocery store, like Publix, Sweet Bay, Akins or Whole Foods that carry a wide variety of organic foods, then half the battle is won. If not, it will take some driving around to find all the foods you need. This is more of walking the walk; so, don't give up!

Another great place for fresh fruits and produce is your local farmer's market, where farmers bring their produce in trucks and sell on a certain day of the week. Hopefully, your local health food store is going to carry plenty of organic foods and staples for you to complete your list through the rest of the week.

Another good find is a well-stocked vitamin and supplement store where you'll be able to quickly and easily pick up your supplies. The specific supplements you'll need are listed in chapter 7, so please refer here for a complete list of supplements for fighting breast cancer. If you are diagnosed with any other type of cancer or you are using this book as a foundational tool, contact a doctor of Naturopathy or nutrition specialist for the correct supplements to benefit your individual battle.

If there is anything you can't find in the stores, shop the internet. If you are not yet shopping online, I suggest you get comfortable because it is fast, convenient and all-inclusive. I have listed some good websites in the last chapter. If you find a product online that you really like, research the ingredients and dosage. Check the quality and quantity, and choose products that have the ingredients you are looking for without a lot of extras added. The internet can save time and money, and you can cross-reference the products to find the best bargains and sales. Bookmark your favorites for quick reference, so you don't lose them.

As time went on, I began to get to get to know the people in the stores that I frequented around my home, which helped immensely when I had questions. They either knew the answer or they knew where to send me for more information. The demand for live, healthy foods is growing rapidly, so you'll find many delicious foods as you transition away from dead foods. They may even be foods you have never tried before, and that's good.

Keep walking the walk and talking the talk. Don't give up, and don't give in. Remind yourself over and over again - " I am a winner; I'm healthy and cancer-free. Nobody can tell me anything different! I'm healed from the inside out, and I trust in God."

Remember All Water is Not the Same

One of the most important steps in forcing the malformed cells out of your system is to drink water, lots of water. Check back to Chapter 5 for the details. By instinct, I knew I should be drinking filtered or bottled water, but did you know that the different brands of bottled water are actually filtered to different degrees? That left me wondering which brands were better because I usually just bought whatever was on sale. Bottled water is not the best choice, but we all need it in the mobile world we live in. I had to find a better solution for clear, clean water.

So, I took a giant step in my recovery walk and made an appointment to have the city water tested at the house. When the representative showed me the water coming out of my kitchen faucet, I couldn't believe it was so dirty! Have you ever seen the sediment and residue that are in your public water system? It is horrible! I was totally disgusted because I knew this was average city water, and it was contributing to the malformed cells in my body. I knew by looking at it that no one should be drinking that water. This water wasn't going to flush out any cancer cells, in fact, I think it was contributing to the disease. Needless to say, I installed a reverse osmosis filter as soon as I saw what I had been drinking.

This turned one of the best things I have ever done. I added a filter for the shower, and if you don't have either, I suggest that you find a good brand and seriously consider the reverse osmosis filter. Install it on the kitchen faucet, and you'll have clean water for drinking, cooking and washing your foods, which is so important. I couldn't believe the amount of water a person uses in a day until I began to monitor my water intake to flush out the malformed cells. You can't carry cases and cases of water into the house every other day, and the reverse osmosis is a much more efficient filter.

The high quality of a reverse osmosis system far exceeds the filtration of the average bottled water. Consider it an investment, in yours and your family's health. It will last for years, too.

While shopping for the right filter, chose Aquafina, SmartWater or an alkaline water like Waiakea Hawaiian Volcanic Water in bottles because these have the best filtration. When you're in the fight and for optimum health, you need to drink at least 8-10, 8-ounce glasses of water per day, so you have a continual flow of crystal clear water washing the toxins and impurities out of your body. You can't do it with Coca-Cola, Kool-Aid or alcohol. These are foods that cancer cells consume to multiply.

Summary

So far, it's not too hard, is it? Read the labels – no sugar, flour, chemicals, hormones or steroids, and especially no aspartame. No foods with preservatives might seem impossible, but if it's not real food, don't eat it! And, five ingredients or less on the package is what to aim for. If there's more, that's fine. Always keep in the back of your mind that millions of people prefer this diet, so it must be good. The biggest incentive is if I can do this without my chocolate chip cookies and Pralines and Cream ice cream every night, you can too! This is our life we're talking about!

Follow-up Appointment or Not?

So, by now your follow-up appointment has been scheduled, and the time has arrived to draw the line in the sand. Here is where courage and confidence step in because unless you have an extremely lenient doctor, they will be expecting you to go forward with their treatment schedule. They may give you a month to make your final decision, and after that, they will have to terminate the relationship. There are physicians who will cooperate and maintain a watch over you, but not many. My doctors wouldn't monitor my progress, and it felt like I was going against the entire AMA when I told them that I had decided to go with holistic healing instead of the surgery, radiation, and chemo they had planned.

It is very difficult to go against the system. Most of us have put doctors in the position of gods, never daring to question them. Then when something like cancer hits and they don't have all the answers, you realize that they are only human and there are other options available. It's up to you.

So, what was going to be the best way for me now? Being a baby boomer and coming from a somewhat non-traditional mindset, I think I was somewhat prepared for this. Doctors aren't perfect in my eyes. They have their place, in testing and procedures, but ultimately, they work for us! This is MY LIFE, and I have come to believe that I have a choice in the type of treatment I choose to submit to, and all of the evidence points to healing from the roots instead of treating only the symptoms.

When I was 10, and I needed a penicillin shot, my parents took me to the doctor. As I was leaving, they would hand me a lollipop for being good. Think about it. They were keeping the sugar-disease concept alive, thereby ensuring my return for another sickness. But I'm not 10 anymore. I'm older and hopefully wiser, and I can't put my trust in a profession that is not seeking effective solutions for this disease. Doctors are actively contributing to a death rate that is spiraling out of control, and I know I'm worth more than that, and you are too.

When I got to my doctor's office, I was determined to remain tactful because I knew in a year, or less, that I would want an MRI to prove my healing. By the Grace of God, I had moved and it was funny, the six-month checkup was arranged by my new gynecologist. I did not even need the assistance of the original doctor.

It felt really good to talk to my new doctor about my program and what I had been doing to treat the cancer. In these six months, I had gained so much information; everything I'm sharing with you. I felt confident that I was doing the best thing for myself using natural methods to eradicate the cancer cells and bring my body back to good health.

The most important thing that I now realized was that I wasn't alone. I had switched my healing strategies from a death-oriented medical one to a life-oriented supportive one, and it felt fantastic to walk right out of the office! When I left the doctor's office, I headed to my health food store to find something nutritious to celebrate with. My how things were changing for the better.

Chapter 11

God, Why is this taking so LOOOOOOOOOONG??

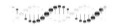

I mpatient? Of course, you are. What is the timeline for healing when you can't see anything happening? Waiting with absolutely nothing visually or physically changing on the outside is extremely frustrating, but we are building faith, and here we are.

At times, it felt like I was watching my fingernails grow. Then I would turn over and watch the dust collect on the table; lay on the sofa and do breathing exercises, repeating over and over again how grateful I was, trying to stay positive by speaking that all the malformed cells were gone, and God had healed me from the top of my head to the tips of my toes. I pictured all the things I was going to do as a healthy person, and I was not including those people in my everyday life who always had something negative to say about my condition. Remember, actions and reactions will follow your thinking and speaking, whether it is positive or negative. Only the consequences will change.

When you have wounds on the inside and you can't see the progress, it is only the hope and faith that keeps you from going insane and helping you do the next right thing. You've found the best ammunition: the right supplements, drinking liters of water to flush the deformed cells out and eating nutritiously for the fight is pulling out the heavy artillery.

In some cases, you just have to wait for the miracle to happen by being determined not to give up. Remember, many others have been through this process and have emerged Victorious, and I know if I can do it, then you can too!

Inside the Hula-Hoop

The human part of us asks questions such as "What is going on?" "Why didn't somebody tell me before that I was killing myself with those donuts and diet soda?" I know they said I'd get fat, but no one ever said anything about contracting diseases like cancer!

The truth is if it falls inside my hula-hoop, it's my responsibility. The hula-hoop only fits one, me, but I have full control and responsibility for everything that concerns me. Even if a friend calls and says they want to go shopping, so we do and my wallet gets stolen from my purse while we are walking, I can't blame it on her because it was my choice to go with her, I need to make the right decisions to cover myself.

So, I am responsible for my hula hoop, and you get to do the same. Make decisions, feed, rest, take care of in every way – yourself. Don't let the opinions of others change your decisions for health and well-being that you have already made, and use the word prevention wisely. The Father says "Wait, slow down" especially when you're not sure of the next right step. Keep doing the next right thing.

It's amazing how everybody in the house is now willing to eat whatever Mom is cooking, even if it's healthy! They are actually learning good, healthy life skills that will make their lives better in the long run. They are learning to choose the right foods and to eat less junk food, which is the secret to preventing disease at the roots. Children who learn a clean and natural way of eating at a young age will be positively changed for the rest of their lives. When the cycle of unhealthy eating is broken, the family can enjoy better health for generations to follow.

What's Happening? – I'm Encouraging You!

For those who are in the fight, I'm sure frustration and aggravation have seeped into your thinking, but look at everything you've learned in this short amount of time! When you have finished this book, you will have learned incredibly sensible and healthy ways of shopping, cooking, exercising, resting, preparing fresh, nutritious juice, and you will have discovered how to release stress and anxiety while helping your family to be at peace too.

Changing your lifestyle 180 degrees can be extremely frustrating because everybody wants it to happen yesterday. But, you didn't Get sick overnight, so becoming adapted to a healing lifestyle won't happen overnight either. It is a process of replacing old behaviors with new ones, little by little, bit by bit, during the natural occurrences of the day. But if you stick to it, change does occur and you'll begin to see healing begin to take place.

Keep doing the next right thing; juice some carrots, beets, cabbage, and spinach, a great antidote in combating malformed cells and sagging thoughts. Things are going to get better if you keep at it. Turn it over to God to handle; He's got the solutions.

This is war; and every time you can add some more powerful antioxidants for more ammunition, you are doing something productive. Hit 'em Hard! Pick up the Word, and read it daily for inspiration along with any other positive literature you can find to keep your thoughts full of light. God loves you more than you will ever know, and He's got a plan for your life!

What's so Funny?

One of the best antidotes you have in your arsenal is laughter! You say, "what is there for me to be so happy about?" Laugh at ANYTHING – it doesn't matter, but keep fighting the fight with all the laughter you can muster. Laughter is known in many healing circles and hospitals as being the Best Medicine. The Word says it is! Endorphins are released and stimulated to move throughout your system with good, hearty, belly laughs. Research has found that the more the endorphins are aroused and released, the more they encourage healing, while also lifting your spirits and keeping depression away. Who doesn't want that? So laugh.

- The effect is similar to the effects of serotonin and dopamine, two additional hormones in the brain that must be at the proper levels in order to get a good night's sleep.
- Laughter encourages the immune system to perform better, which then affects your entire body, promoting healing. So don't stay sad or filled with gloom – LOL. Make time to Laugh Out Loud every day!
- Go to your local movie rental and pick up some comedies, knee-slapping, funny movies where a belly laugh is inevitable. You may end up laughing for an hour. Find the humorous sitcoms and cable

comedians to lift your spirits, and don't spend a lot of your time watching the news. There will always be bad things happening, so let's just ignore it for a season.

From time to time you may think you are losing the battle because you feel tired or fatigued, but it is only natural to get worn down when you've been fighting. Ask any soldier, and you are a soldier in the army of "kicking out disease and taking back good health!" So, put away your worry and fear, take more naps and allow your body to eliminate malformed cells while you sleep. You were made to win. So, think like a winner and you will be a winner!

The last golden nugget: Don't be concerned with the days on the calendar and the hours in a day. Time is not in our hands, it's in God's, and He says that a day is like a thousand years, so who's going to count? His thoughts are higher than our thoughts, and His ways are higher than our ways, so we rest in His work and do the next right thing.

All things will happen according to His incredible timing – stay aware. This is your time to do the things you have procrastinated for years such as putting your old photos together in a photo album, cleaning out the drawers or emailing and writing friends and family that you haven't heard from.

Learn to make new nutritious, delicious dishes or create a new juice. Don't get stressed out and don't overwork yourself, but if you're not staying busy, you're going to get bored and depressed.

Here a gratitude tip:

Imagine if you had not been introduced to this healing way of life, and you only had the traditional methods to treat your cancer? You would feel terrible, depleted and fatigued all the time, but you are killing off the malformed cells and replacing your good cells in a combat where the good wins, all while restoring your soul with spiritual food and rest for recovery. So grateful.

Chapter 12

April Showers Bring May Flowers and Summertime

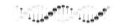

Finally, as the longer days and warmer temperatures begin to come out, life begins to show more promise, and the pace appears to pick up. I began to feel better after the winter months were over, and the added daylight was helping my attitude too. Who would've thought that living naturally and nutritionally could make a person feel so good? It's amazing what happens when you really put your heart and soul into positive change. I wish I'd learned this way of life 30 years ago. The positive literature I've been reading, getting healing words into my spirit and releasing all the built-up stress is giving me a new perspective on life. Surprisingly, I like trying all the new foods I have to choose from in recovery.

I have been looking forward to seeing progress. I've been waiting patiently like the rest of you have for the day when they can test the amount of cancer that is in my body. I'm sure most of you are much stronger than I am, and you have chosen to put the disease behind you and walk forward. I'm not looking back, but I want to see the test clear and cancer-free. The time has arrived for my six-month follow-up diagnostic mammogram. To say I was anticipating the results is an understatement. I called the hospital and made the appointment.

After six months, I had gotten really good at juicing, and I hope you are, too. Fruit and vegetable juicing bring back memories of when I was in my twenties living in Miami. We would juice wheatgrass into small, shot glasses and down the "instant energy." Wheatgrass supplies amazing nutrients that provide intense energy with only a small amount of juice. It's power-packed, but you can get a similar energy boost by juicing carrots, spinach, and other greens, and they offer such super support for the immune system.

In six months, I have totally changed my diet to alkalizing my system with fresh whole foods. I have come to rely on my AM and PM breathing exercises to remain calm and peaceful through the day and to have some quiet time to talk to my Creator. I have had no pain whatsoever, just slight fatigue from time to time.

In fact, I'm feeling better and better, so I know I am winning this battle. My body knows that it has been in a strenuous fight, and I know it too. There have been many who are praying for me, and I know that My God shall supply all my needs according to His riches in Glory. It's easy to see how much Father God cares and loves us. Just look around and see how He gave us courage and determination to fight this evil disease day in and day out. His mercies, His Love are new every morning and as His children, He'll never leave us. He always loves you, and He'll never leave you alone. He becomes more to us as we grow closer to Him.

Section Especially for Women in Menopause

My appointment was set for July 22, and I now know what Tolstoy meant when he said, "It was the best of times, and it was the worst of times." In hindsight, this has been the story of my life. In October 2007, I turned 50 years old, need I say more to the women — when it rains it pours.

Women reading this section will know exactly what I mean with one word - menopause. Just to clear the record, I have been going through perimenopause for about five years now. I would've thought it'd be over by now. I didn't want to take HRT, hormone replacement therapy, synthetically, so I have been building my hormones back naturally with soy products, Black Cohash, which also acts as cancer suppressant, yam supplements, and bio-identical progesterone.

If you are a woman, it is vital for you to use either a natural or synthetic HRT program. You can look at menopause like Dr. Braverman in New York: He says that Menopause is actually the death of the reproductive system, so a hormone regime is needed to maintain your system. If you do nothing, it will not function properly and slow down and you'll have no energy. I recommend the natural; it is simple and everything you need can be found at your health food store.

As you age, male or female, the hormones decrease, but they are vital to your system, to keep you looking and feeling young. I first began using progesterone cream, which is made from yams. It is a topical cream that you apply to the skin, like your stomach, and it is absorbed into your system. I also drank a soy protein shake every day, but research has shown that 95 percent of the soy today is GMO produced, so you will have to either find a soy powder that is 100% organic or use a whey or plant-based protein powder. As I said before, protein is in every cell of the body, so it is vital to supply your body with a premium protein every day. There are many excellent brands available today.

It might help your understanding to research soy for yourself and read the differing opinions. Some sources report that it is 100% GMO or scientifically produced, but if you search, natural soy protein is available. Natural soybeans with soy isoflavones can be very helpful for females because science has proven that soy produces estrogen, a female hormone. Tofu is another option.

For this reason, soy products are not recommended for men. The benefit is to reduce the many menopausal symptoms including hot flashes, which were almost non-existent for me. Men need other hormones replenished such as testosterone, and these come in supplements also. The combination I used for about five years worked wonders in calming and smoothing the emotional ups and downs that drive women crazy. Use soy in moderation, and if you're not sure if it's organic or not, check the label. My hormonal experience going through PMS with high quality, natural supplements was much easier than the stories I heard from my friends.

Try naturally building your hormones, but if you decide you don't like it or it doesn't help after two to three weeks, just stop; there will be no side effects because you are using all natural supplements. But, if you are at this point in your life, you need to address your declining hormones in some way because hormones motivate your entire system to work optimally, and you need the best performance possible for cancer-crushing. The hormone system can be effectively and easily regulated with natural and bio-identical products.

Two other supplements that contributed to reducing menopausal symptoms are Evening Primrose Oil and Cat's Claw. These worked really well with the natural progesterone cream specifically reducing hot flashes and mellowing out the hormone imbalance. You will need to work through this season of your life, but it will get better when once you are treating it with effective supplements.

Consult your gynecologist, and the two of you can decide on what HRT treatment you'll use. There are some great, natural bio-identical hormones including progesterone, testosterone, estrogen, and thyroid hormones, so there's no need to take synthetic ones. If your gynecologist is not knowledgeable about natural treatments, go online and take the information you find into your health food store and ask them for assistance. A naturopathic doctor would have this information also.

More and more female gynecologists are reaching outside the medical box obtaining knowledge in natural supplements and incorporating it into their practices. It would be absolutely phenomenal to have all physicians step up and learn the value of natural supplements, but this isn't going to happen anytime soon.

My Six-Month Mammogram

So on July 22, I got in the car and drove back to the hospital where I had gotten the initial report of multifocal cancer in my right breast six months earlier. I hadn't been back since then because of their uncooperative attitude of alternative methods of healing. They had given me only ultimatums, including forcing me to return in 30 days or risk being discharged and not one doctor offered to monitor me throughout the process.

All of those involved in the medical community said the same thing, including the surgeon at the hospital where I was headed. "No Guts" these guys and no stamina. How did they ever get into their profession? I'd like to think that when they were younger they might have been more flexible, but now the consensus seems to be conformity to the same sorry standard procedures that have used for over a century and a half.

I was somewhat apprehensive as I was driving, but it was a familiar route, so I tried to think about other things. I had been looking forward to this day ever since I began experiencing the success of this program. I was eager for some visible results. I had been working so diligently at improving my immune system and kicking out the cancer that I wanted to see how much the cancer had decreased. I wanted to show the entire medical profession that healing occurs outside of their watch. If I had to wait another six months, so be it. There are no timetables with God, but I really wanted to see a cancer-free report!

It's time that alternative healing methods were acknowledged and accepted outside the medical profession because more people are dying than ever before to cancer and other diseases of immune disorders. Traditional procedures simply aren't working.

I'm almost to the hospital, which is on a barrier island on the coast of the Atlantic. Every room in that hospital has a huge picture window view of the bay. It's one of the most beautiful hospitals I've ever seen, but I won't be staying there. I walked into the Women's Center and in an hour I walked out. They would send the results to my gynecologist. Since I had my nutritional routine down by now, I just continued with what I had been doing. It was out of my hands.

I felt so good that I started doing some volunteer work that week. I hadn't worked in my profession for over 8 months, so it felt good to get out in the community.

Fourteen days later, I went to my gynecologist for my office visit and the results of the mammogram! I was also expecting the results of a vitamin and mineral deficiency test from the gynecologist, so this appointment would be interesting. I recommend these vitamin levels be tested at least once a year. They are covered by most insurance policies for that time period, and they include a liver and thyroid test, in addition to the levels of vitamins and minerals in the blood. It is the liver that does the work of eliminating the toxins and cancer cells from your body, and the thyroid gland regulates the hormones in your body. Hormones, like serotonin, affect the brain's activity, and estrogen and progesterone work together to support the female body to balance the other hormones.

Men, this change of life applies to you, only in just a slightly different way. You would need the same tests, but your hormones will be different - definitely minus the estrogen, of course. Your doctor can order these tests for you. Let them know that you are interested in learning about the decrease of hormones as you get older, And how you can supplement that. If they cannot suggest any natural alternatives, try your local supplement store or health food store. Hormone levels are important to a properly running body, so don't neglect them.

Back to my office appointment; Dr. Shepard walked into the office and saying, "MY MAMMOGRAM CAME BACK CLEAR of all CANCER!!! I was CANCER-FREE! Miracles do happen! I was ecstatic and beside myself! Literally! The fight was over, and I knew that thousands of people could benefit from the way I had washed the cancer out of my body, and the knowledge I had gathered to reach this success. I couldn't wait to get back home and tell everyone I knew!

I knew I was going to be sharing my journey of success, so I scheduled an MRI in January 2009, exactly one year from my diagnosis. Perfect, it was exactly the proof I wanted to have.

In the following weeks, I read information on mammograms, and research has discovered that they contribute approximately 10% to the development of new breast cancer, so now I use MRIs or ultrasounds instead of mammograms. After all, I'd been through, I did not want to go through it again, and it's as easy as a simple request to your doctor when you make your appointment. Most insurance plans cover the alternates.

Chapter 13

This is a Fight, Not a Dance!

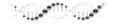

Cancer, more than most diseases, has to be treated aggressively because it's roots go deep down to affect the whole person, mind, body, soul, and spirit. Cancer turns fatal when the host refuses to acknowledge all of these doors to their complete healing. When they go untreated, the multiplication of the malformed cells increases. So, even if the original tumor was found in the breast, the entire body is actively trying to evict the intruder cells of cancer, before it metastisizes.

No one who has been diagnosed can sit around and wish their cancer away. Deciding not to go the traditional route for treatment means that you are going to attack the disease and fully participate in your healing. If you choose chemo and radiation, you'll take an equally active role in restoring your good cells that were annihilated when the chemicals and radiation were applied. To restore your body back to its actively functioning state means you'll need to take this book in hand and commit to the fight of restoration from the serious side effects that these two archaic methods produce.

If you have decided to use traditional methods, the information in this book will be equally as life-changing for you as well. This program and the nutrients and supplements that are needed to fight cancer will likely reduce the time and the symptoms by building up and re-establishing the cells and tissue that have been destroyed after each treatment. Medical doctors typically order tests throughout the treatment to determine the amount of cancer in your body, and by using the tools I have laid out, the recovery will not be as drastic, traumatic or destructive as it is with people who don't have this vital information.

Chances are that by using this program, you will be back to better health much faster because the tissues will receive the benefit of having complete nutrition to support the healing. If you eat junk food and donuts during this time, your body can not receive the necessary nutrients that it must have to recover. In fact, there is a good chance that continuing to eat sugar-filled foods and bread will prolong the treatments. You can't eat whatever you want despite what the medical team tells you.

Never let the disease think you are getting complacent or you're thinking of giving up on your recovery because that will only allow the cancer cells to multiply at a tremendous rate. Never let this disease gain a day in your recovery plan. Stay on top of it. Yell, if you have to, but never give up on seeing yourself healed. This is a fight between the good cells and the bad. Cancer has no place in any life on this planet, and with determination and diligence, you can evict it and be cancer-free again. God is Good – All the Time!

Chapter 14

The Turnaround

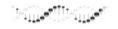

This is called the Turnaround chapter because in one year my life completely turned around for the better, and I have proof. It has been one year since I received the diagnosis of multifocal breast cancer and the prognosis for a double mastectomy; that was on December 27, 2007. Everything has turned 180 degrees; nothing is the same as it was. I look healthy, I feel healthy and I am now 100 percent confident that God is alive and cares about me and the details of my life. I have the results from my MRI that was taken in July 2008, and THERE IS NO TRACE OF CANCER IN MY BODY!! AMAZING!! A Miracle!!

There is no reason to fear cancer, malformed cells or the diagnosis of any other disease that might try to attack me. I am a cancer survivor who has overcome cancer with a scientifically sound, natural solution that was fueled by the power of the Creator of the Universe, and you are with me on this journey. The plan is to eliminate the cancer cells from your body because they don't belong there. They are invaders and must be evicted.

Unbelievers

I showed the results of my MRI to the four doctors I contacted for the second opinion after the diagnosis. I wrote letters to each one and spoke directly to the original surgeon, and they explained away my healing as "luck." They were not interested in the treatments I had used to attain this success. I thought they would surely want to know more about alternative treatments to save the lives of their clients, but they didn't. I couldn't have been more disappointed.

They did not want to acknowledge success outside the narrow statutes of the AMA, though the United States is losing patients to cancer at a rate of 1 in 3. The medical community is losing the fight, and there are more solutions. I don't understand it. When there is an answer, why can't the medical authorities and insurance companies at least acknowledge the information and techniques and cover according to the success rate? I was extremely disappointed with their reactions, but if they listened to my story of how I overcame cancer, then they would have to deny treating the symptoms that the medical treatment stands for, and that is their livelihood.

Believers

On the other hand, the orthopedic physician I had for over 20 years listened intently as I explained what I had been doing the past year, and he embraced the whole program. Also, my gynecologist was extremely excited with my program and the results, but she already uses nutrition, natural vitamins, and supplements in her medical practice. She has established an optimal support program for women who want to be able to explore all of their options whether alternative or traditional. She is a forerunner for her profession, and if there were more medical professionals that followed her example, the medical system in America would be turned upside down; thousands of lives would be saved every year. The medical professionals in your life have to be informed when you show them your cancer free test, so slowly, they will accept the alternatives more readily.

Share this Book Freely.

Today, I am still eating, drinking and living very close to the way of eating I designed during my year of recovery. This lifestyle is a process that prevents all kinds of diseases, in addition to cancer, from overtaking me. Vitamins, minerals and other nutrients are necessary for a healthy lifestyle because the food source and the environment are only getting worse. Our lives before this plan was detrimental to our health, look what happened!

Maintaining an alkaline system to prevent and cure diseases along with the other food concepts in chapter 5-7 will allow you to maintain a lifetime of better health with more energy. I hope and pray that if you retain anything, it is that toxic foods only create havoc and destruction in your body, and sugar is cancer's best friend, so it is your worst enemy!

When you receive the cancer-free declaration from the physician, you can begin to add other foods, but be careful what you add. Check them out to make sure they fit the standards of non-toxic foods and introduce them slowly.

My regime of supplements changed slightly after I was not in the fight any more. I discontinued Healthy Cell, IP-6, the Killer Mushroom, Cat's Claw and Black Cohash, but it will be a lifetime of adapting and adjusting the supplements I need for every season that I go through. But, that's OK, I have a healthy lifestyle now that allows me to be flexible, while still maintaining structure and discipline. I added glucosamine/chondroitin/MSM to strengthen my joints, but these are individual choices you can make for yourself at any point.

The most extravagant change that has occurred is that now I have a sense of confidence and I am happy and full of joy. I feel freedom from the bondage of sickness that held me captive. I know that God is always on my side, and I can count on Him; He releases all the stress that comes my way.

I have learned to forgive and forget, most of the time. Life is too short to carry unforgiveness and offenses around like a bag of rocks. I've let the heavy cloud of disease go, and I want to stay walking on the care-free path of life. Sure, there are going to be other problems down the road, but I know there's nothing that my Father, the Healer, and I can't handle together. My part is to do the next right thing and be obedient to Him. Love surrounds me and you too, when you ask Him too.

I hope and pray that your success comes to you quickly. Remember, there is no turning back – you're on the road to victory now. Be well and be blessed, and at all costs, relieve stress, forgive others, stay alkaline and laugh until it hurts! Keep this handbook to refer to and grow from, and to share with others. We shall surely meet on the road of our Joyful Destiny.

I have lived these instructions and was told to share the path with everyone exactly how it happened. Overcoming cancer presents a tremendous challenge in God's children, and I would like to invite you to share your testimony if you would like. My email is at the end of the book.

Now, give the life-saving information you have to someone who needs it. Buy a book for them and be a life-giver in this journey. I am looking forward to the destination one day, and I want to take as many people with me as possible. Won't it be spectacular to meet others who overcame this evil enemy while we were on Earth. Our lives were increased and improved and we got to live longer and better! God Bless you!

Read Again!

Chapter 15

Recipes and Websites

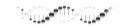

T his chapter was added to offer a glimpse at how to get started on this healthy way of living with some recipes for daily living, but let creativity be your guide when preparing healthy meals. I have included easy, nutritional recipes that fight cancer and are just plain delicious and nutritious.

Below are Some Favorite, Cancer-killing, Immune-building, Natural, Organic Recipes for use every day.

Abbreviations for recipes below: c = cup; t = teaspoon; T = tablespoon

- My Favorite Smoothie

1 c. Almond milk or
½ c. Almond milk and ½ cup juice (pineapple or apple are good)
1 banana
1 t. cinnamon

Add your choice of fruit into a blender: 4-5 strawberries, a small handful of blueberries or/and 10-15 red grapes or blackberries, orange pieces; all are packed with anti-oxidants to feed your immune system.

Add a handful of fresh spinach and one scoop of vanilla whey protein powder, which adds 15 - 25 grams of protein per scoop depending on the brand. Use a brand with no added sugar or sugar substitute and no preservatives or chemicals. Label should show sugar is less than 5mg.

Blend all until smooth.

Add 6-8 ice cubes, one at a time. Pour into glass and Enjoy! A protein smoothie is a nutritious way to start the day or have as a mid-morning/mid-afternoon snack. The protein will satisfy you for 3-4 hours. Don't have one close to bedtime because your body will be detoxing as you sleep, and protein is more difficult to digest.

- Sweet and Sour Salad

Wash and drain well one head of Romaine lettuce. Cut into one inch pieces and place in large bowl. In a separate bowl, whisk together – 1/3 c. Raspberry Vinegar, 1/4 c. olive oil. Salt and ground pepper to taste.

Slice one cucumber and add to the cut Romaine. Pour dressing over salad, toss and mix. Add a can of mandarin oranges, drained, and arrange on the salad mixture. Sprinkle with your choice of walnuts, pecans, almonds or sunflower seeds. Voila' - a quick, delicious snack or partner to a meal.

P.S. The nuts give your salad "staying" power with protein. Add three ounces chicken breast or wild salmon, broiled or grilled, for a complete meal.

- Juicing

Juicing is super important to the fight, and it is super easy. If you are in the fight or want to infuse nutrients into your system effectively, juicing is super-packed with vitamins, minerals, flavonoids and other nutrients that your body needs. Nowadays, it's possible to find fresh fruit and vegetables year-round, so juicing is convenient every day.

To start making your own fresh juice, all you will need is a good juicer. This appliance extracts the juice from fruits and vegetables separating the seeds, peel and flesh from the juice. They are available in retail stores or online ranging from $19.95 to $400. I recommend selecting one in the mid-range price, so you get a well-built machine that will not too expensive or difficult to use. Shop around before you purchase, so you can see the differences. Walmart and Kmart have some efficient juicers at reasonable prices, but you'll find many other reputable brands in other stores that carry products for the home.

Purchasing the juicer is the hardest part! Making your own delicious fresh juice is fun and extremely healthy! The energy and benefits that come from juicing are incredible, and you can create such a large variety of flavors. Make your own favorites anytime for a delicious glass of juice, and it will be in your system in 20 minutes or less.

In juicing, the vitamins and minerals are released at the very moment the juice is released, so you want to drink it immediately. When you cook vegetables, some of the vitamins and minerals are lost, so by juicing, you are supplying your live cells with the pure nutrition they need to overcome and kill the cancer cells. The benefits of juicing far outweigh any prepackaged, concentrated or even organic, low processed juices because fresh juice is pure and completely absorbed by the body. Juicing is the super-nutritious way to feed every good cell in your body.

Here are some favorite juicing recipes:

Immune Building 1

Juice 5 carrots, ½ medium beet, ½ Granny Smith apple, a wedge of cabbage and a handful of spinach. Add ½ medium peeled cucumber. Pour into a glass with or without ice. Squeeze ½ lime or lemon by hand to top it off. Enjoy!

Immune Building 2

Juice 3 tomatoes, handful parsley, 2 cloves garlic, ½ peeled cucumber, 2 celery stalks, 1/8 onion and 4 carrots.

Alkaline Special
¼ head cabbage, 3 stalks celery, ½ peeled cucumber

Liver Tonic
4 carrots, ½ medium beet

Chlorophyll Cocktail – Bring on the Greens
5 carrots, handful of spinach leaves, handful of collards
or Kale, 4 sprigs watercress

Blood Regenerator
6 carrots, handful of spinach, ½ medium beet, 4 parsley
sprigs, ½ Granny Smith apple

Digestive Tonic

6 carrots, handful of spinach and/or kale, ½
peeled cucumber

Body Cleansing
Use Digestive Tonic recipe and add 1 medium beet

Health Heart
5 carrots, 3 broccoli florets, ½ inch slice fresh ginger, ½
Granny Smith apple

Juicing Tips:
- Have at least 6-8 oz. of fresh-squeezed juice twice a day.
- Lettuce is 99% water, so don't bother juicing it. Make a salad instead for the fiber. Juice spinach and kale, for better results.
- Put carrots in large end first. This prevents jamming.

- Fresh juice begins decomposing and loosing vitamin potency about 20 seconds after it is juiced, so drink it right away. It cannot be stored long.

Enjoy making fresh juice for your friends and family anytime, but it's a requirement when fighting the fight.

- Natural or Organic Pumpkin Recipes

It is always the perfect time for pumpkin - natural, pure pumpkin. Pumpkins are a member of the squash family, and therefore, very good for you nutritionally, plus it adds a rich flavor to protein smoothies and yogurt.

Pumpkin, whether fresh and cooked or canned, is an excellent source of manganese, vitamin C, copper, magnesium, vitamin A, dietary fiber, potassium, folate, and phosphorus. In addition, summer squash is a good source of omega-3 fatty acids, vitamin B1, B2, B3 or niacin, B6, calcium, zinc, and protein.

With all these nutrients packed into pumpkin, let's find some ways to get this great vegetable into everyday meals. Below are some delicious recipes that you can enjoy year 'round with natural canned pumpkin, which is delicious and has no artificial ingredients, flavors, additives or preservatives.

For a quick snack at night or in the morning, try natural or organic pumpkin mixed half and half with natural, unsweetened applesauce with a sprinkle of cinnamon on top. Add yogurt, chopped pecans or walnuts for added protein. Naturally sweet and delicious!

Pumpkin Milkshake

In a blender:
    1 c. Almond, soy or rice milk
    1/3 c. pure canned pumpkin, not pumpkin pie mix.
    1 scoop vanilla whey protein
    ½ banana
    Strawberries, red grapes or two slices fresh pineapple for sweetness
    1/2 t. vanilla
    ¾ t. cinnamon

Blend until smooth. Add 6 to 8 ice cubes and blend until smooth. Pour into tall glass and garnish with a sprinkle of cinnamon. If you desire, add ¼ cup Ezekiel 4:7 cereal. Enjoy!

Pumpkin/Raison Yogurt

    In a small bowl:
    Start with 1 c. natural or organic Greek or Goat's milk yogurt (no sugar or additives)
    ½ c. pure pumpkin
    ½ c. unsweetened applesauce
    ½ t. vanilla

Sprinkle cinnamon and nutmeg to taste.

add 1/3 c. raisins

Stir to mix. Chill. Sprinkle with walnuts or pecans or Ezekiel 4:7 cereal. Tastes like a chilled pumpkin pie! Enjoy instead of ice cream or sugary desserts. Great for breakfast too!

- Healthy Alkaline-producing Recipes

Everyday Salad

Wash and drain well one head of Romaine lettuce. Cut up into 1" pieces and put into large bowl. Add: one Zucchini sliced/cut in half, 1 small onion sliced, 6-8 sliced white or Bella mushrooms, 1 sliced hard-boiled egg

Sprinkle 3T. EVOO (Extra virgin olive oil) over the salad. Then sprinkle with Balsamic or a flavored Vinegar like Pomegranate Balsamic. Grind fresh pepper over the top to taste. Toss. Sprinkle with ¼ cup Sunflower seeds.

Alternative: add 1 sliced sweet potato! Yum!

Tip: use EVOO on salads and cold foods, and use Olive or Grapeseed oil to cook with because they have a higher smoking point than EVOO.

Simple Tomatoes and Rice Refrigerator to table in 20 minutes.

Ingredients needed:
    Rice or Ezekial Pasta - follow directions for cooking.
    1t. Balsamic vinegar
    3 T. Olive Oil
    2-3 cloves of chopped garlic
    small onion, chopped
    sea salt and fresh ground pepper to taste
    1 lb. sliced mushrooms - Baby Bellas have extra flavor!

To the side:
    2 Tablespoons fresh Basil, julienned, thinly sliced.
    5-8 Heirloom or Roma tomatoes, chopped or use 2 cans of petite cut tomatoes.

Add vinegar, olive oil, garlic and onions to a medium skillet along with sliced mushrooms. Sautee lightly for 3-4 minutes then add tomatoes. Save the Basil to add two minutes before you are ready to serve. Pour complete pan over a bed of whole wheat rice or Ezekiel pasta. Serves 2-4. Sprinkle lightly with Parmesan cheese.

Cabbage Soup – Yummmmm!

In large soup pot: always make a pot full, so you'll have plenty of leftovers when it's twice as good!

Add ½ c. olive oil to a large pot. Add one chopped onion, 4-5 garlic cloves minced, 4-5 stalks of celery chopped, and one green, yellow or red pepper sliced thin. If y ou like peppers add a variety of colors. Sauté' five minutes on medium heat.

Core and slice one head of cabbage to 1-inch pieces. Add to pot and stir.

Add 4 cans or 2 boxes of organic Chicken or Vegetable Broth. You can always add more while cooking to make the stew/soup as thick as you like. Put the cover on, and bring to boil; simmer for 10 minutes.

At this point, you can add any combination of vegetables that you want. Fresh is best, but frozen is equally as nutritious. Here are some ideas: Broccoli, cauliflower, diced tomatoes, green beans, spinach, kale or other greens, carrots, peas... Every time you make Cabbage Soup, it will be different!

Add tomato juice, if you want a tomato-type base. Simply use equal amounts of stock and tomato juice.

You may NOT use corn OR any variety of beans such as black beans, kidney beans or pinto beans if you are fighting cancer. There is too much sugar conversion that occurs in these during digestion, but they are still good and healthy for the rest of the family. I like to add brown rice. So add one cup of rice directly into the pot, along salt and pepper. This recipe makes a huge pot that you can use as side dish or soup.

Feel free to add whatever herbs you like, the more the better as they are packed with healing properties. Oregano, Thyme, Basil, Rosemary, Sea Salt or Italian herbs are favorites. Now that everything is in one pot, turn down to low and let SIMMER. The longer it simmers – the better tasting the soup will be, but you can serve it in about 20 minutes. Spoon into bowls and sprinkle with Parmesan cheese.

Simple Caesar Chicken Pasta Salad

Ingredients. Mix in one bowl:
  2 c. thinly sliced Romaine lettuce
  1 ½ c. cherry tomatoes – halved
  2 t. thinly sliced fresh basil
  ½ c. chopped green onions into ½ inch pieces
  2 garlic cloves, minced
  1/3 c. oil and 2 T. balsamic vinegar mixed for dressing
  ¼ c. chopped fresh parsley

1 – 4 oz. pkg. crumbled organic Feta cheese

Add:

3 c. skinned, boneless, shredded roasted chicken breast – still warm.

3 c. Ezekiel 4:7 Penne Pasta (about 6 oz. uncooked) – still warm.

Combine all ingredients in a large bowl; Toss gently to coat. 4 servings.

Wheat- free Pasta Puttanesca

Pasta Puttanesca is a typical "old Italian" dish, but by making it wheat-free, it will not be typically Italian. But, the sauce is delicious and will taste authentic and 'old' school.' The Puttanesca recipe goes back to the mid-1900's when the brothels of Italy were "state-run." The name actually means 'pasta, the way a whore would make it' or a 'whore's pasta.' The ingredients are simple and easy to find in the grocery store and to keep in your pantry for a last minute dinner.

Traditionally, Puttanesca would be served with fresh pasta, but since this is a wheat-free dish for cancer fighters, try using whole grain rice, spaghetti squash or Ezekial 4:7 pasta; rice noodles could be used, too. Check in your local health food store if you can't find any in your local grocery and keep these ingredients on hand.

Sauce:
   1/2 cup olive oil
   4 cloves garlic, finely chopped
   1 c. sliced mushrooms
   1 small onion, sliced very thin

Sauté lightly in a large skillet. Add:
   2 cups chopped tomatoes; fresh or two cans of petite cut.
   4 anchovy fillets, rinsed and mashed with a fork
   2 T. natural tomato paste
   • 3 T. capers
   • 20 Greek olives pitted and coarsely chopped
   • ½ - 1 t. crushed red pepper flakes, depending on taste.

Let simmer on medium heat for 10 minutes. At the end, add chopped basil leaves and cook two more minutes. Then add cooked noodles and toss lightly. Pour into serving dish and if using rice, first spoon rice into a large bowl and pour sauce on top. Add parsley and parmesan to garnish.

This will become a favorite for family and friends alike. Easy to prepare and delicious to eat, so enjoy your wheat-free Puttanesca!

- Incredible Eggs

Keep hard-boiled organic and natural eggs in the refrigerator at all times for quick access. For hard-boiled eggs, take eggs from refrig to come to room temperature; place eggs in pan and cover with cold water. Place on stove, and bring eggs to boil, then reduce heat to low and cook for 15 minutes. Remove from heat, and run cold water over them for several minutes to chill. This reduces the dark color around the yolk. Refrigerate.

Basic Omelet:

Preheat skillet with olive oil and butter. Lightly sauté whatever veggies you like for 3-5 minutes: such as mushrooms, peppers, onions, garlic, grated zucchini, broccoli, spinach, kale, whatever you like.

Crack 3 organic eggs in a bowl. Add a few T. of water/milk and whisk well. Add salt and pepper. Pour over sauteed veggies and let cook thoroughly. Serve with salsa and 1 or 2 slices Ezekiel bread and tea. Butter is good, do not use substitutes. Good Anytime!

Two eggs over easy cooked in a skillet coated with olive oil and butter with two slices Ezekiel bread is a great, go-to breakfast!

Spaghetti Squash – is the fun squash! Cut in half lengthwise and scoop out the seeds, not the flesh. Spread olive oil along the inside and place face down on cookie sheet.

Bake at 425* for 25 minutes. Take out and let cool 5 minutes or until you can hold it. Then take a fork and "scrape" the inside until it is completely shredded. This is the spaghetti-like look, and It is excellent to use this in exchange for any pasta recipe you have.

Quick Tomato Sauce

In a side pan, sauté 2 cloves garlic and 8 oz sliced mushrooms in olive oil. Pour in 2 cans of petite cut tomatoes; add salt and pepper, basil or your own favorite spices for unique flavors. Let simmer for 10 minutes and pour over spaghetti squash. You can add veggies, if you like.

Vegetables are so versatile. Add them to everyday meals for additional nutrients and value. Be creative and mix the colors!

Natural Foods are fun, nutritious and full of flavor! You will feel so good eating these whole foods. Mix and match in new ways, remembering to use a rainbow of colors for best nutrition. Create new dishes that you might never imagined before with these junk foods.

GLOSSARY

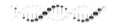

Benign - a mild type or character that does not threaten health or life; especially, not becoming cancerous as a benign tumor - having no significant effect: harmless.

Cancer - Cancer begins with one cell that divides and reproduces abnormally and then continues to multiply with uncontrolled growth. These malformed cells can break away and travel to other parts of the body, setting up another site or metastasis. Growths and tumors will grow from the cells gathering together.

Chemo - Chemotherapy is the use of drugs to kill bacteria, viruses, and cancers, which inevitably kill all cells, whether good or bad.

Gynecologist - a physician with a practice centered on the care of women.

Malignant – means "to produce death or deterioration" as in cancer, which infiltrates, metastasizes, and appears fatal; a malignant tumor.

Mammogram – is a certain type of x-ray, which detects tumors in a woman's breast before she can feel them. Used regularly for cancer detection.

Metastasis - the spreading or transferring of cancer cells to other areas of the body.

Multi-focal breast cancer – means "many points" so, in this type of cancer, there is not a lump present, but many smaller lumps. Multi-foci means that the cancer cells are forming in strings throughout the tissue like pearls.

Natural foods – foods that are whole, having no chemicals or preservatives.

Oncologist – doctor who specializes in cancer treatment using surgery, radiation or chemotherapy treatments.

Organic foods – foods that are completely free of chemicals, steroids or preservatives in every way including how they are grown, processed and shipped.

Radiation – a treatment for cancer using the process of emitting radiant energy in waves or particles to attack the malformed cells.

Supplements – a naturally made food or vitamin added to fortify one's diet.

Vitamins – any naturally occurring substances essential in certain quantities to the body for both human and animal.

References:

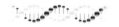

New Living and King James Bible Bible.com or GatewayBible.com

Romans 8:28 All things work together for the good of those who love the Lord and are called according to His purpose.

Matthew 6:33 Seek first the Kingdom of God and His righteousness, and all things will be added to you.

John 10:10 The thief cometh only to steal, kill and destroy, but I have come that you may have life and life more abundantly.

John 3:16 For God so loved the world that He gave His only begotten Son that all who would believe in Him might be saved.

Isaiah 53:5 By His stripes, I am healed. He was wounded for our transgressions, He was bruised for our iniquities; The chastisement for our peace was upon Him, and by His stripes, we are healed.

Luke 1:37 Nothing is impossible with God.

These are websites I found to be very helpful.

- www.whfoods.com Here is an excellent website for learning exactly what vitamins and nutrients are in foods. You can check which foods have more antioxidants, vitamins A, C and E and all the other nutrients. Remember, the more antioxidants the better as they battle the free-radicals.
- When making menus, try to use a rainbow of different colored fruits and vegetables. The different colors specify different nutrients and levels of nutrients, and you'll find an incredible variety of reds, yellows and greens. The Rainbow Diet and Rainbow Recipes is a book written by the Bravermans, which will offer delicious natural recipes.
- The Maker's Diet is a diet and collection of recipes based on what humans were originally created to eat. Both The Rainbow Diet and The Maker's Diet are very informative and will help you create

new, healthy, naturally-nutritious meals. They are both available online.

- www.elook.org/nutrition/herbs is a web page on herbs that is invaluable. Herbs are an easy way to add extra nutrients and super flavor to meats, salads, and veggies along with salt and pepper.

- For more information on foods to make your system alkaline, google "alkaline foods." You'll get hundreds of articles on alkaline foods along with many useful charts.

- www. Puritan.com is a nutritional online whole-sale store where you can find most of the supplements mentioned in this book.

- www.barleypower.com - barley adds alkaline to your system, so, if you are finding it difficult to keep your system at the 7.2 – 7.6 ph level, take 4-6 Barley capsules every day. This company produces quality capsules.

And national websites on cancer:

The Truth About Cancer, T.T.A.C.	-	thetruthaboutcancer.com
American Medical Association	-	www.ama-assn.org
National Cancer Society	-	www.cancer.gov
American Cancer Society	-	www.cancer.org

Postscript

This manuscript is an outpouring expression from my heart to you who have been afflicted with the disease of cancer. It was my privilege to write my experiences in this handbook as God told me to do, so I could share my successful pathway.

I have ventured to tell the entire story of the one year of my life after diagnosis with all the honesty and attention to detail as I possibly could. I tried to include everything because I know that different, individuals hear and learn from different segments, but rest assured, I attempted to transfer the words God gave me, so your lives would be touched by Him.

Your journey is equally significant, and together if we share our stories freely, more people will become survivors and be able to call themselves Cancer Overcomers, like you and I, in the years to come.

After, a decade as a Cancer Overcomer, I have made incredible progress in becoming the person that God wants me to be. This season was turned from evil into a starting point. I believe that it was through this journey from the darkness of this disease into His Healing Light that doors opened within me that I never knew were there.

It was not the destination that had so intrigued me, but the journey of hope and grace that I now find every single day as I walk through my life sharing my faith in God.

Hopefully, you can identify with me and be transformed out of death into a marvelous Life and the struggles that are included. This disease is cunning, baffling and powerful, and it affects all the feelings, emotions, and situations that we struggle with as humans. There is no other disease or sickness that compares to it.

Recovery means so much more to someone who has been given a death sentence, but who found that the journey allowed them to discover the essence of their lives and who they really are - spirit, soul, and body.

This is our promise from God for eternity to come. "I know the thoughts that I think toward you, says the Lord, thoughts of peace and not of evil, to give you a future and a hope." Forever. Jeremiah 29:11

I am so excited to have published this book, and that you have read it! God gets all the Glory! In the following months if your life has changed, I would love to hear what happened and how you feel today. God is really Good; All the Time! Please send your testimony to LizGamble7@Gmail.com.

Testimony from Amy M. -

Diagnosed with breast cancer in 2008, I began to eat and pray like God would want me to. Psalm 103: 1-5 is my favorite scripture. I was encouraged and strengthened as I learned of this natural journey of healing that I used for recovery along with surgery that removed the tumor.

Today, I continue to remove the toxins from my diet, drink kale smoothies, and I eat a rainbow of fresh, raw vegetables with low sugar intake. I am blessed with a blended family of four boys and two grandchildren. My day starts with prayer, meditation, and scripture to help me focus and trust in the Lord for my daily needs. I'm very grateful I learned how to be healed with this natural process.

Jesus is the same yesterday, today and forever.

Jesus is the same yesterday, today and forever.

Jesus is the same yesterday, today and forever.

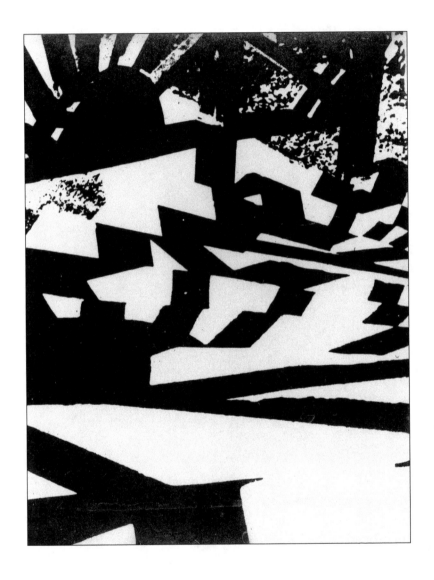